A Colour Atlas of
Clinical Operative Dentistry
Crowns and Bridges

Second Edition

J. Ralph Grundy
BDS, (B'ham), LDS, RCS(Eng), MDS, VU(Manc)

formerly Senior Lecturer and Tutor in
Conservation Techniques, University
of Birmingham Dental School,
Consultant Dental Surgeon,
Birmingham Area Health
Authority (Teaching)

John Glyn Jones
BDS,(Lond), LDS, RCS(Eng), FDS, RCS(Eng), PhD(B'ham)

Senior Lecturer in Restorative Dentistry
University of Leeds Dental School,
Honorary Consultant in Restorative Dentistry
United Leeds Teaching Hospitals
NHS Trust

Wolfe Publishing Ltd

Second Edition Copyright © 1992 Wolfe Publishing Ltd
Published by Wolfe Publishing Ltd, 1992
Printed by BPCC Hazells Ltd, Aylesbury, England
ISBN 0 7234 1724 5
First edition published in 1980.

A CIP catalogue record for this book is available from the British
Library.

For full details of all Wolfe titles please
write to Wolfe Publishing Ltd, Brook House,
2–16 Torrington Place, London WC1E 7LT.

Contents

Preface to the Second Edition

Since the first edition of *A Colour Atlas of Conservative Dentistry*, some 11 years ago, there have been many alterations and modifications to the practising techniques of dental surgeons. This, in conjunction with developments in the field of dental materials, has necessitated the radical rewriting of some sections of the book. In particular, the current management of early caries has led to considerable revision of the concepts of cavity preparation, with a greater emphasis being placed on the preservation of sound tooth tissue than has previously been the case. In addition, the inclusion of a new chapter that covers the monitoring and maintenance of restorations has been considered appropriate with the knowledge that, again, a more conservative approach should be adopted in the evaluation of existing restorations.

Greater emphasis can now be placed on the role of adhesives in modern dentistry. Considerable advances have been made in this field during the decade since the first edition was published, with the advent of porcelain veneers and a wider use of minimal preparation bridges, both now accepted as viable treatment options.

Whilst it is recognised that clinicians will have their own preferred material and methods of execution for many of the clinical procedures discussed, we have attempted to illustrate broadly the various techniques available in the belief that these can be adapted by any operator for any given circumstance. It is the principles involved that are important in ensuring that a satisfactory result is achieved. This approach will be appreciated especially in the chapter devoted to impression techniques and the authors hope that, by this means, the book will be of value to undergraduates and clinicians with all levels of experience.

Finally, again no attempt has been made to render the book definitive in its own right. This would be too presumptuous as excellent texts, many of which are included as recommended reading at the end of the volume, already exist on the various aspects of conservative dentistry. It is hoped, however, that the atlas will fulfil a valid function in that the illustrations will bring pictorial impact that words alone are unable to impart.

Preface to the First Edition

The title [of the First Edition], *A Colour Atlas of Conservative Dentistry*, implies something more than operative dentistry but less than restorative dentistry. For instance, patient assessment, plaque control, crowns and bridges are included, whereas periodontal surgery and the provision of dentures are not.

It is hoped that the Atlas will provide vivid graphic support for dental students, embellishing their clinical experience, and also offer some fresh views and ideas for qualified practitioners. The latter might use some of the pictures to explain certain forms of treatment to their patients. It is not claimed, however, that this Atlas is in any way a testimonial to the dental paragon; indeed a number of less than satisfactory outcomes to treatment are included to stress that all practitioners of this most exacting art, conservative dentistry, experience difficulty, on occasion, in achieving perfection!

Although some aspects of the author's philosophy on his specialty are included by way of introduction, the Atlas is designed predominantly to be complementary to the many excellent textbooks on conservative dentistry and not to be a complete text in its own right. Pictures in this Atlas have been chosen where they might illustrate points better than black and white pictures found in the standard textbooks. Where appropriate, references are made to some of these textbooks and to the dental literature so that when read in conjunction with the Atlas, a full description of each topic may be obtained.

Acknowledgements

The authors are, once again grateful to their colleagues for readily granting them access to collections of photographic material in the search for clinical examples and for allowing those selected to be included in this edition. For this, appreciation in particular is expressed to Mr PB Begley, Mr M Cassidy, Mr DM Martin, Mr BR Nattress, Mr CJW Patterson, Mr SL Pearson, Dr CG Plant, Mr JP Ralph and Mr CC Youngson for allowing us to use pictures from their personal collections and to the staff of the Department of Medical and Dental Illustrations of the University of Leeds, Mr AJ Robertson, Mr DA Hawkridge, Mr P Parkinson and Mrs Mary Lunn, for undertaking much of the clinical and non-clinical photography; Mr PH Newsome and AE Morgan Publishing Ltd., for permission to reproduce figures 268, 269, 270 and 271 which were first published in Restorative Dentistry; and Drs L Trondstad and TI Leidal, University of Oslo, for permission to use figures 178, 179 and 180 which first appeared in the *Journal of Dental Research*.

Figures 402, 540, 545 and 602 were first used by Dr J Glyn Jones in *The Dentition and Dental Care*, (1990), and permission to reproduce these has kindly been given by the Editor, Professor RJ Elderton.

Several pictures have been carried over from the first edition and our thanks are once again due to the following - Mr AS Britton, Professor RM Browne, Dr JC Davenport, Dr FJ Fisher, Professor AR Grieve, Dr MC Grundy, Mr N Hall, Mr PS Hull, Dr MA Mansfield, Mr DK Partington, Dr WP Rock and Professor DS Shovelton. Figures 553 and 555 (previously 408 and 410) are used with the permission of John Wright & Sons, Bristol and appeared in *Inlays, Crowns and Bridges*, Ed. Kantorowicz (1979).

The authors are indebted to Professor A.R. Grieve for his preliminary advice and constructive comments following the preparation of the text.

We wish to thank again Dr J C Davenport, and this time also his daughter Sarah, for their artistic skill in providing artwork in addition to that which Dr Davenport provided for the first edition.

Mr M Sharland and Miss M Tipton of the Photographic Department, Dental School, University of Birmingham, are to be thanked for taking several clinical pictures and for copying many others.

Finally our appreciation must also be recorded to our students and patients. The former for undertaking some of the clinical work selected for illustration in the Atlas, and the latter for their forbearance in allowing the necessary photography to prolong their treatment sessions. We sincerely acknowledge their co-operation.

1 Patient assessment and treatment planning

Before starting any restorative work, it is sound policy first to assess the patient as a whole person. Identical clinical conditions are not necessarily treated in identical ways and a multitude of factors will be influential in the formulation of a treatment plan. Not least amongst these will be the patient's wishes, availability for treatment, age and general health.

The mouth should also be regarded as a whole before work is started on a single unit within it. Diseased teeth may be treated in a variety of ways, and the condition of the other teeth and the supporting structures can determine a definitive treatment plan.

Not all diseased teeth require treatment. Much will depend on the individual oral environment and the influence brought to bear on this by the society in which the patient moves. A well-motivated patient living in a sophisticated society, supplied with fluoridated water, with access to fluoride toothpaste, dental floss, and regular dental checks, may well be given the opportunity for any small carious lesions to arrest or re-mineralise. Recurrent caries at a defective filling margin for such a patient can possibly be prevented from progressing and the guideline for the dentist should be 'if in doubt wait'; rather than, as in years gone by, 'if in doubt, fill – or refill'.

At the other end of the social scale or in countries without sophisticated dental services the dentist should not strive officiously to restore every diseased tooth when the patient may prefer to avoid heroic restorative treatment and await multiple extractions and full dentures.

In order to consider quickly and efficiently the multiplicity of factors that influence dental decisions it is advisable to have a set procedure for recording a *history* and undertaking an *examination* (see Appendix 1) in order to aid a thorough dental assessment.

Full information obtained from such a comprehensive scheme of enquiry and observation will allow the formulation of a *treatment plan*. This may vary considerably for superficially similar dentitions and it should not be assumed that there is a standard form of treatment for each manifestation of dental disease. For example, for a patient with extensive caries, the treatment plan may be to remove the carious tissues and restore the teeth with the best filling materials available. On the other hand, for a patient who has ineffective or poorly motivated oral hygiene, it may be necessary to make a two stage treatment plan. The first part aiming to establish good oral hygiene, with the second part being dependant on the outcome of the first - success leading to advanced restorative work and failure to basic minimal restorations or even extractions. Thus, the patient's motivation is a critical factor in determining a treatment plan. In this context it is useful to employ a Plaque Index or a Gingival Index, which can give a numerical value to progress made in oral hygiene improvement. This can be of help in developing the patient's motivation, especially in association with a disclosing solution enabling the patient to monitor progress at home.

Although this Atlas deals mainly with the conservation of teeth this must never be considered in isolation to the neglect of other specialities. In the concept of treating the mouth as a whole, the need for a patient to undergo orthodontic or prosthetic treatment may lead to a decision to extract a tooth although it is capable of restoration. Simply because it is technically possible to restore a tooth does not mean that the tooth must be restored.

Interrelationships between specialities must also be appreciated. The design of a partial denture may influence the design of restorations if the incorporation of rest seats, retentive undercuts or guide planes are necessary.

Many personal factors can modify a treatment plan, for example, the availability of the patient to attend for a lengthy series of appointments. Whilst the ideal treatment plan might include the provision of crowns, bridges and inlays, the patient may be unable to find the time or the money for this advanced work to be undertaken. The time involvement and the cost could therefore be reduced by restoring the smaller lesions with amalgam or composite, extracting the teeth needing more complex restorations and replacing them with partial dentures. The possible permutations within a treatment plan are too numerous to list here but a few general principles are given as a guide to priorities:

- The treatment of pain must take precedence over all else.
- Teeth of doubtful vitality or with extensive carious lesions should be thoroughly investigated before a definitive treatment plan is established. Large lesions should be stabilised at an

early stage with temporary dressings so that the lesions do not progress whilst waiting their turn for treatment.

- Scaling, polishing and plaque control should precede all other treatment, except for pain control and stabilisation, for the following reasons:

  (a) It gives the opportunity for the patient's motivation and effectiveness in plaque control to be monitored during subsequent treatment sessions.

  (b) The patient's response to plaque control may necessitate modification of the rest of the treatment plan.

  (c) Being comparatively unintrusive and painless, scaling and polishing is a good introduction to a course of dental treatment and helps to establish a good operator/patient relationship.

  (d) The improvement in appearance and freshness of the mouth following this phase of treatment can raise the patient's interest in, and appreciation of, dentistry.

  (e) It often results in a more pleasant mouth for the dentist to work in.

  (f) To facilitate operative dentistry - for instance, by a reduction in gingival haemorrhage, by revealing the true shade of the teeth for accurate colour matching, by establishing the true gingival margin before teeth are prepared for crowns, and by the removal of calculus to allow the proper application of matrix bands.

  (g) The need for periodontal surgery can be assessed.

- Where a partial denture and restorative work are both required, the denture should be designed before restorative work is started but the restorative work should be completed before impressions are taken for the denture.

2 Plaque

For any particular patient, the amount of plaque retained on the teeth can vary considerably according to the interrelationship between dietary intake and the frequency and effectiveness of the plaque removal methods employed. Whilst it is not intended that this book should act in any way as a text on Preventive Dentistry or Periodontics it must be emphasised that effective plaque control is a prerequisite for the successful restoration of teeth. In this endeavour, it is important for the dentist to be able to monitor the plaque state of the mouth. Such monitoring is more meaningful to the dentist and dramatic for the patient if it can be measured and recorded, and there are several plaque and gingival indices that can be used for this purpose.

An important criterion of an index to be used for an individual patient, as opposed to one for use in epidemiological surveys, is that it should be easy to employ and be capable of giving an overall 'plaque picture'. One plaque index (Appendix 2) is the Patient Hygiene Performance (PHP) of Podshadley and Haley (1968). The significance of any plaque index will of course be influenced by the time interval since the patient last cleaned their teeth, and this must be borne in mind in discussions with the patient.

The PHP index, however, only records plaque deposits on selected teeth whereas the Hygiene Index (HI) proposed by O'Leary *et al.* (1972), evaluates all tooth surfaces by means of a yes/no decision for the presence or absence of plaque. It is therefore a simpler and more comprehensive demonstration of tooth cleanliness.

For recording gingival inflammation, indices have been developed which are based on the registration of a single characteristic of gingival inflammation, for instance bleeding on probing, (Ainamo and Bay, 1975). Scoring is performed for all tooth surfaces and can therefore indicate a percentage of gingivitis in the mouth. The Community Periodontal Index of Treatment Needs (CPITN), was reported by Ainamo *et al.* (1982), and combines clinical findings with treatment needs.

1 The gingivae seen here are as near-perfect as can be achieved with the conscientious use of plaque control methods. The gingivae meet the teeth in a 'knife-edge' margin, the contour of which follows the amelo-cemental junction around all the teeth. The interdental spaces are well filled and the gums are light pink and show stippling.

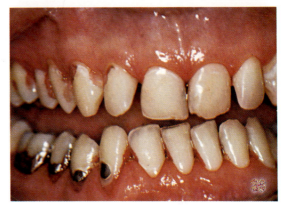

1

2 Most surfaces of the teeth of this patient are free of plaque but a disclosing solution reveals very light deposits which might otherwise have gone undetected, particularly interproximally in the upper right quadrant and lower incisor region.

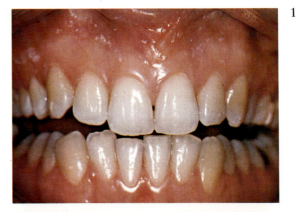

2

3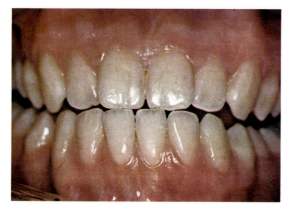

4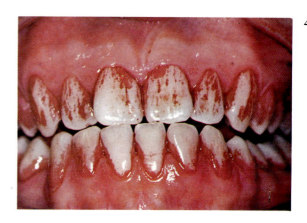

3, 4 Without the aid of a disclosing solution the plaque deposits on these teeth are barely detectable. Occasional slight signs of gingival inflammation indicate where deposits might be (**3**). After the use of a disclosing solution, widespread plaque deposits against the gingival margin are revealed (**4**).

5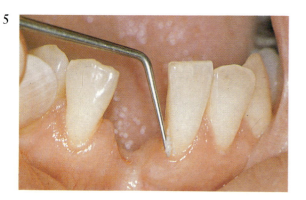

6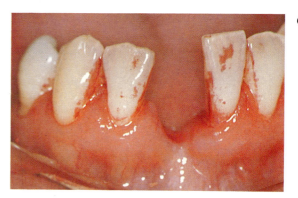

5, 6 A thin film of plaque near the gingival margin is detectable by running a probe across the tooth surface (**5**). The plaque is however better seen by both dentist and patient with the more sensitive method of applying a disclosing solution (**6**).

7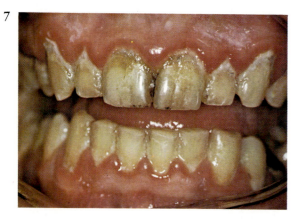

8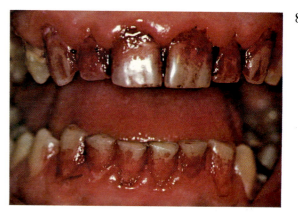

7, 8 These gross plaque deposits near the gingival margin are obvious to the naked eye (**7**) resulting in generalised marginal gingivitis. This is recognised by the 'rolled' gingival margins, the swollen interdental papillae due to the oedema and the reddening of the free gingivae due to hyperaemia. The use of Neutral Red as a disclosing solution is recommended more to shock the patient than to inform the dentist (**8**).

9 Heavy deposits of calculus are usually seen without recourse to disclosing solutions as on the lingual surfaces of the six lower front teeth. The heavy staining, possibly by tobacco, tea or coffee, indicate that the deposits are longstanding ones. It is important for the dentist to remove this calculus so as to allow the patient access to the teeth to keep them free of plaque deposits by home care. Smaller deposits of unstained calculus, matching the colour of the teeth, are readily revealed by the air spray. This not only reflects the gingivae to give a good view into the pocket but also dries the calculus turning it to a chalky appearance which contrasts clearly with the shiny enamel.

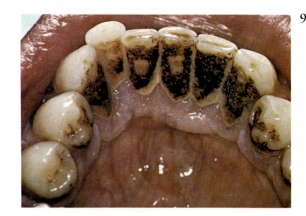

9

10 The complete absence of any oral hygiene in this mouth is emphasised by the layers of desquamated epithelium left undisturbed on the attached gingivae.

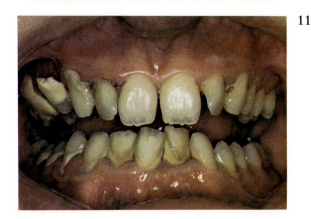

10

11 This patient has exceptionally heavy deposits of calculus on both upper and lower teeth on the right but no obvious deposits elsewhere. This condition is brought about by the avoidance of chewing on the right side and should warn the dentist to look for some underlying cause.

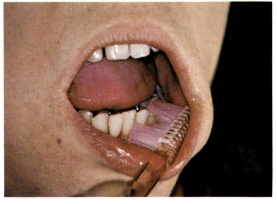

11

Plaque control

12–16 Following the removal of all deposits from the teeth, it is essential to guide the patient in methods of plaque control if rapid re-deposition is to be prevented. Ideally, before any course of conservative treatment is started, the patient should demonstrate their toothbrushing technique (12). This should be improved by advice from the dentist when it is found to be inefficient and checked at subsequent visits throughout the course of treatment.

12

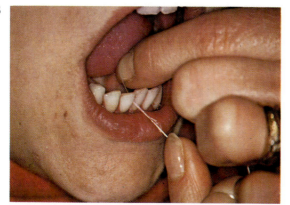

Interproximally, the teeth are not usually accessible to the toothbrush. Where there is evidence that plaque is causing inflammation of a papilla, the interproximal tooth surfaces can be cleaned by dental floss (13) which wipes off the plaque deposits from each tooth in turn. The floss may often be more easily controlled if it is first wrapped round each middle finger and then eased between the contact points with the index fingers.

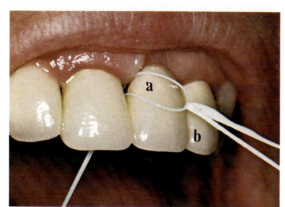

Where there is difficulty in introducing dental floss, for instance between the retainers and the pontic of a bridge as seen here (14), it may be assisted by a floss threader, a stiff strand of nylon with a loop (a) at one end. The floss is first threaded through the loop (b) and the threader is passed, stiff end first, through the gap pulling the floss after it. The floss threader is reusable if washed. Superfloss also has a stiffened end to aid its insertion and may be easier to use than a floss threader, but is more expensive than standard floss.

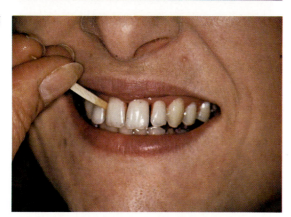

It is possible to use a wood stick interproximally where there is space to introduce one (15). Patients often find sticks easier to use than floss but being straight and rigid, they do not clean convex surfaces as effectively. Concave, interproximal surfaces pose problems for both floss and sticks. The answer in such instances is to use the bulkier end of Superfloss.

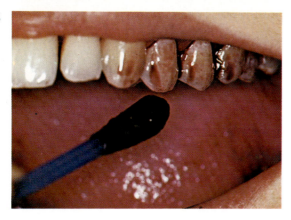

At regular intervals, the patient should monitor the effectiveness of his plaque control by the application of a disclosing solution (16). Food dyes are cheap, nontoxic and readily available. After thoroughly cleaning the teeth, the disclosing solution is applied with a cotton bud by the patient and the excess rinsed away. The dye stains any remaining plaque and so shows the patient areas where greater attention is required. A small disposable dental mirror is essential to enable lingual aspects to be checked.

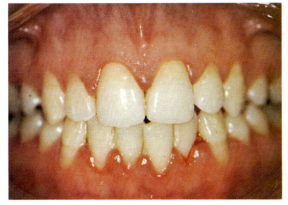

17

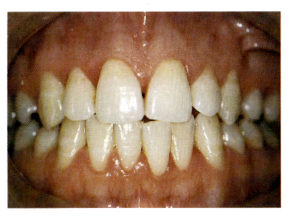

18

17, 18 The benefit of proper home care of the teeth is demonstrated well by this patient who initially showed marked signs of gingivitis (**17**). Solely by the adoption of plaque control methods, the gingivae were restored to health within seven weeks (**18**).

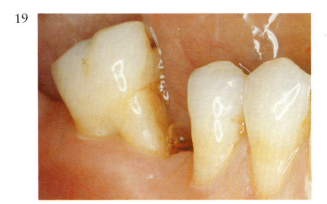

19

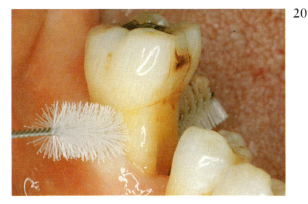

20

19–23 In furcation areas, such as between the roots of this lower molar (**19**), it can be very difficult to introduce floss. Plaque can be removed very effectively from these sites with a 'bottle brush' pushed back and forth between the molar's roots (**20**).

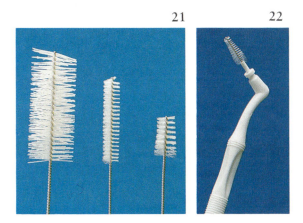

21   22

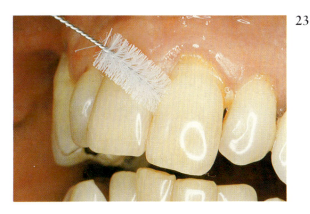

23

These brushes are available in a variety of shapes and sizes (**21**) and some are designed to fit into a toothbrush-like handle (**22**).

The bottle brush also works well in sites where there is considerable gingival recession between teeth (**23**).

24

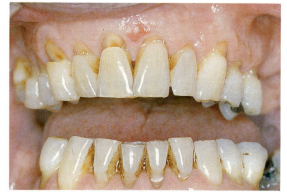

24 Overzealous use of the toothbrush must be curbed if serious abrasion damage to the necks of the teeth, as seen here, is to be avoided. Brushing technique should be corrected by the dentist or hygienist.

25

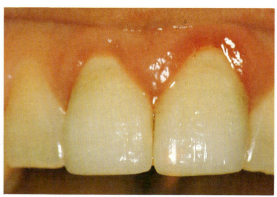

25, 26 Plaque formation may be encouraged by faulty dental treatment; for example, the use of inappropriate restorative materials, or leaving restorations rough, with marginal deficiencies or positive edges creating situations where access for plaque removal is difficult. It is important to realise that faulty dentistry, or lack of proper instruction to the patient can result in soft tissue inflammation where none existed before.

These poorly made porcelain crowns (**25**) have ill-fitting margins making plaque removal difficult. Prior to remaking the crowns, well-fitting temporary restorations should be provided and effective plaque control instituted in order to restore gingival health.

26

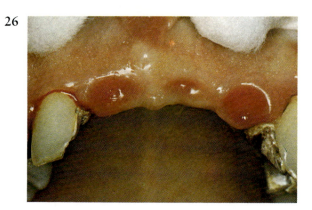

The mucosa under the pontic replacing the upper central incisors and the left lateral incisor was found to be severely inflamed and ulcerated when the bridge was removed (**26**). This was due to a combination of factors. The pontics were made of acrylic which is a material that is badly tolerated by the mucosa - either due to residual monomer or the difficulty in obtaining a smooth surface. Furthermore, the pontics had too broad a contact with the mucosa creating areas which were difficult to clean adequately. It is also possible that the technician 'socketed' the model before making the pontics, a technique which is not recommended.

3 Caries

Caries diagnosis

The gross carious lesion is readily diagnosed by the patient or any other lay person and does not warrant inclusion here. The early lesion however is often far from obvious, especially the Class II interproximal cavity, and careful observation is necessary if such a lesion is to be identified.

The Class II lesion in its infancy is not usually detectable by simple clinical observation unless the absence of the adjacent tooth allows the 'white spot' lesion to be seen. It is therefore necessary to rely on bitewing radiographs wherever posterior teeth are in contact if small lesions are to be diagnosed. Whether such lesions should be treated or simply monitored is a matter of judgement. Often they can be encouraged to arrest or even re-calcify, (see Chapter 8).

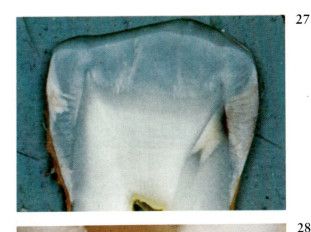

27

27 This stained ground section shows, on the left, an early lesion confined to enamel and probably too small to register radiographically. On the right the carious process, as well as affecting the appearance of the enamel, has also spread at the amelo-dentinal junction and caused a reaction within the adjacent dentinal tubules. There is still no cavitation at the enamel surface and this size of lesion would be the smallest to be detected on a bitewing radiograph (see **38**). This is due to the comparative insensitivity of the radiographic evidence of caries which lags behind the actual lesion (Gwinnett, 1971).

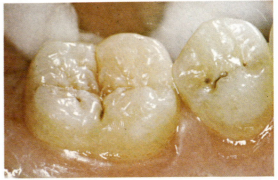

28

28, 29 Premolars and molars cannot be pronounced free from caries by visual evidence alone. These teeth for instance are apparently caries-free (**28**). On bitewing examination however the lower right second molar is seen to have a large mesial carious lesion (**29**).

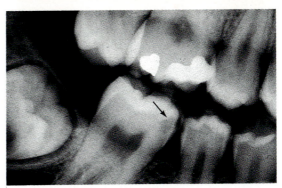

29

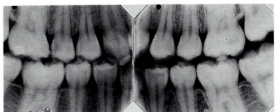

30

30 In purely clinical examination, even dentitions which seem to be totally caries-free can sometimes spring a surprise on bitewing examination, as shown in the upper right second premolar.

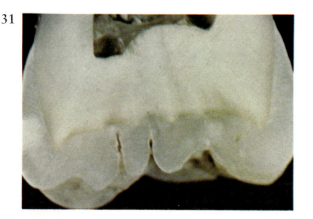

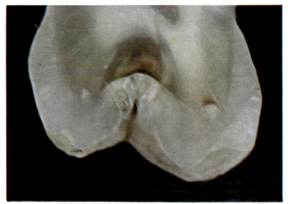

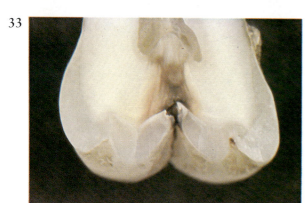

31–33 Class I carious lesions originating in the occlusal fissures of premolars and molars fall generally into three categories. Those where the caries is confined to the enamel (**31**), those where the caries has breached the amelo-dentinal junction causing caries of the dentine (**32**) and those where the caries of the dentine is so extensive that the pulp has been reached (**33**). Clinically each of these situations may look very similar to the naked eye and they may only safely be distinguished by careful inspection of a bitewing radiograph. Nowadays it is not recommended to probe such fissures for fear of either creating a cavity where one did not previously exist or of destroying enamel matrix which might be capable of remineralisation. The modern progressive approach to caries treatment is covered in Chapter 8.

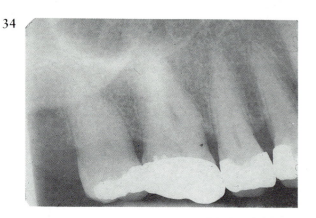

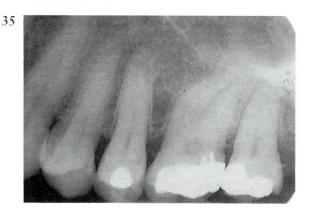

34–37 Bitewing radiographs are preferable to periapicals for caries assessment because, apart from reducing radiation to the patient by reducing the number of radiographs required, the bitewing view of the coronal area is likely to be less distorted than on a periapical film. The distortion however may be reduced by the use of the long cone paralleling technique. A more accurate assessment of bone levels is also possible with bitewing radiographs. These points can be confirmed by comparing the two periapical views (**34, 35**) with

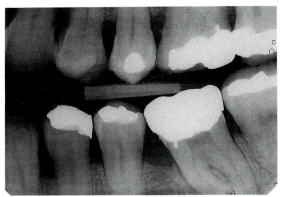

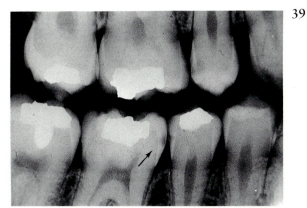

the bitewing radiograph of the same areas (36, 37). As well as detecting caries, bitewing radiographs provide other useful information including, size and position of pulp chamber, interdental bone

levels, quality of interdental bone, existence of amalgam excess cervically, calculus (if deposits are substantial) and the cervical fit of inlays and crowns.

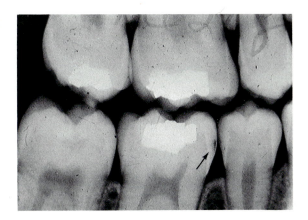

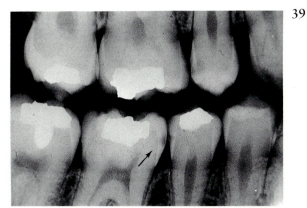

38–40 The rate of growth of an untreated interproximal lesion is very variable. It is reported by Berman and Slack, (1973), as being surprisingly slow. It can however be quite rapid as seen on this series of bitewing radiographs taken at yearly intervals. The lesion mesially on the lower right first molar has developed to a considerable size and a lesion has also started in the adjacent premolar. If any doubt exists about the advisability of filling a minimal lesion it would seem reasonable to monitor its progress at least annually.

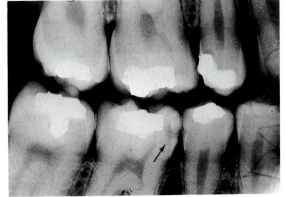

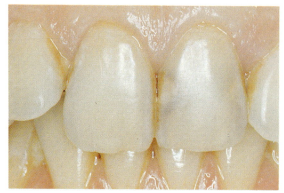

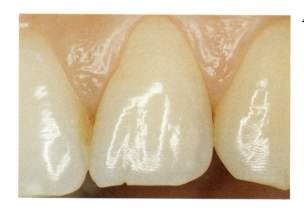

41 42

41–44 Bitewing radiographs are not essential to detect carious lesions in anterior teeth. If a lesion is not obvious in reflected light, as seen mesially in the upper left incisor (41), it may still be detected clinically as these teeth are thin enough to show caries by means of transillumination. In reflected light there is no evidence of caries distally on the upper left lateral in this patient (42). If a bright light is used and the anterior teeth are viewed from the palatal aspect, a carious lesion may easily be seen as a shadow within the body of the crown (43 – arrowed). If doubt still exists the lesion can be shown dramatically by transillumination with a composite curing light (44). It is, of course, necessary to polish off any surface stain before transillumination to avoid confusion.

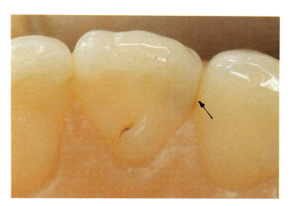

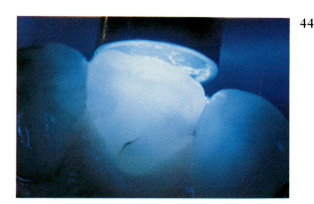

43 44

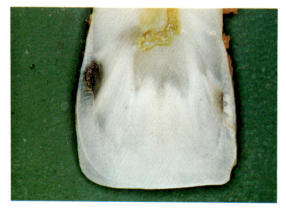

45

45 This sectioned upper central incisor shows a minimal carious lesion on the left similar to the one creating the shadow seen in the previous figure. The lesion has spread at the amelo-dentinal junction but has not yet caused actual cavitation by breakdown of the overlying enamel. Nowadays, if remineralisation was deemed a realistic possibility, such a lesion would be put on probation. The earlier lesion seen on the right might just be detectable using transillumination.

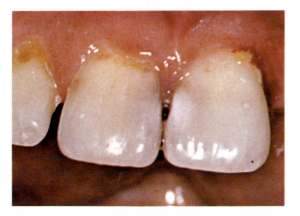
46

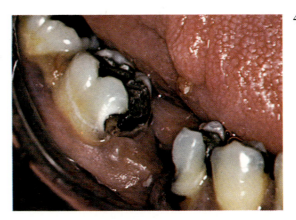
47

46 Larger Class III lesions can be seen by reflected light as is the case with the mesial lesions in these upper central incisors.

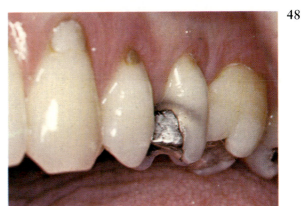
48

47–49 Recurrent caries is readily detected if unsupported enamel breaks away from the margin of a restoration to reveal the carious dentine below, as seen bucco-cervically to the amalgam in the lower right second molar (47). Before the collapse of unsupported enamel, an observant operator can often see the colour changes indicative of carious dentine through the translucent enamel. An example of extensive recurrent caries is shown (48) around the amalgam restoration in the upper left second premolar. The dark banding is due to dentine caries whereas the light discolouration is indicative of secondary enamel caries progressing outwards towards the tooth surface.

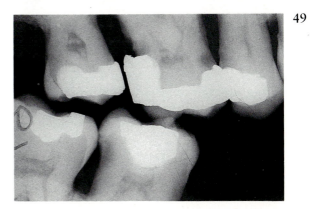
49

Recurrent caries in the depth of a cavity or at the cervical margin may not be seen clinically, although it may be suspected when a history of pulpitis is given by the patient. Bitewing radiographs will often reveal such conditions (49). Here recurrent caries is seen at both mesial and distal cervical margins of the filling in the upper right first molar. Caries is also seen under the Class I filling in the lower right first molar although it cannot be certain whether this is recurrent or residual caries. Primary caries is obvious on the distal surface of this tooth.

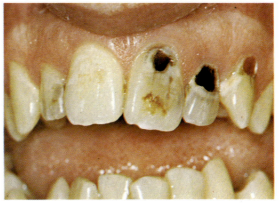
50

50 Unexpected caries confined to a few teeth in the mouth often indicates a specific local factor. The cause of the extensive Class V lesions in the upper left incisors and canine has been traced to mint sweets which were allowed to dissolve slowly in the adjacent labial sulcus.

51

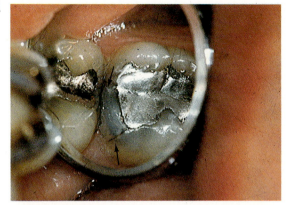

52

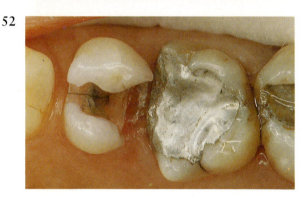

51 A search for caries is frequently initiated by a history of pain obtained from the patient. Occasionally however, a thorough examination fails to discover any caries or exposed dentine to account for the symptoms. A possible explanation may be found in the cracked tooth as seen in the upper left first molar. The enamel shows cracks disto-palatally in two places (arrowed) and these proved to penetrate the full thickness of the enamel thus allowing slight movement during mastication which stimulated the underlying dentine. This 'cracked tooth syndrome', is now recognised as a frequent cause of previously mysterious toothaches (Cameron, 1964 & 1976). Removal of the cracked enamel and replacement with a suitable filling may result in relief of the symptoms if the crack is confined to the enamel.

52 Sometimes the crack involves the dentine and can be very difficult to see. It may be revealed if a curing light is held against the tooth or by the application of a disclosing dye as shown here mesially on the upper left premolar. The pain may be relieved by filling the cavity with a material bonded to the cavity walls to prevent further flexing of the dentine. Further support can be given by a full veneer crown. If the pain persists it may be necessary to remove the pulp in order to save the tooth.

Caries prevention

As well as plaque control and dietary advice, two other methods of caries prevention can be considered - fissure sealing and topical fluoride application. Despite the proven value of both systemic and topical fluoride in preventing caries, it is not as effective for fissured surfaces as it is for the smooth surfaces of teeth. This is because of the difficulties in efficiently cleaning fissured areas. However, a method of overcoming this problem is to obliterate the plaque retentive fissures by filling them with a resin as recommended by Gwinnett and Buonocore (1965).

Fissure sealing

53

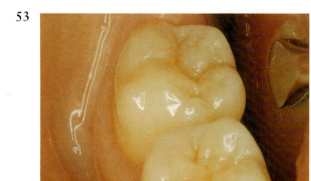

53–61 The lower right second molar shown here is recently erupted and caries-free (**53**). It is considered suitable for fissure sealing.

Its occlusal surface is cleaned as thoroughly as possible with a polishing cup and a paste of pumice and water (**54**) in order to present a bare enamel surface to the etchant.

The etchant gel is applied to both the fissure and the enamel immediately surrounding it (**55**) for 30 to 60 seconds.

After washing away the etchant and dissolved enamel with water, the surface is dried thoroughly and inspected for the frosty enamel surface that

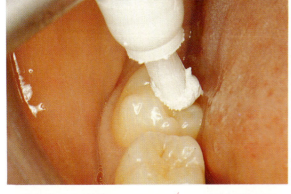

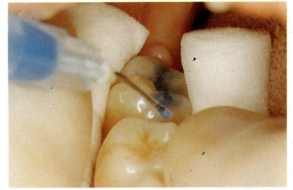

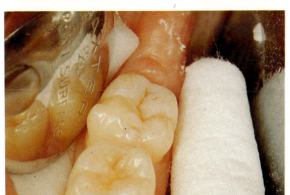

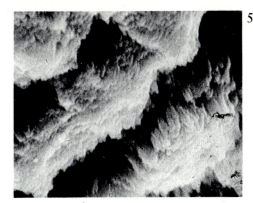

confirms that the etching has been effective (**56**). If this is not apparent the surface should be re-etched.

The effect on the enamel is demonstrated by this SEM picture of an etched enamel surface (**57**). The grossly irregular surface created provides an excellent mechanical lock for the resin. From this point onwards scrupulous moisture control must be maintained if the etched surface is not to be contaminated with saliva, which would interfere with the retention of the resin. If the etched surface is inadvertently contaminated with saliva it must be re-etched before proceeding.

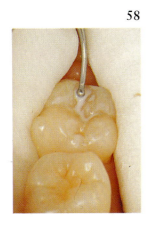

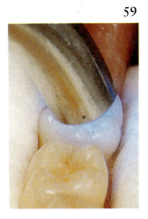

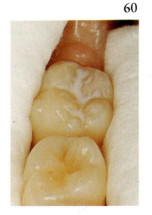

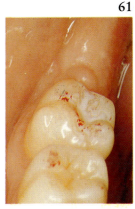

The fissure sealant is applied to the fissures and over the etched enamel using a ball ended applicator (**58**), after which it is polymerised by light (**59**).

Finally, the sealant is checked for completeness (**60**) and, with thin articulating paper, for the absence of occlusal interferences (**61**).

Topical fluoride applications

Fluoride can be added to the enamel surface by topical application, thus increasing the enamel's resistance to decalcification. This can be done daily by the patient through the use of a fluoride containing toothpaste or a fluoride rinse. A boost to the surface fluoride can also be given by the dentist with periodic topical applications of a varnish containing a high concentration of fluoride, such as Duraphat (Woelm Pharma GmbH 3440 Eschwege).

Stabilisation

Caries, being a progressive disease, will extend further into the tooth with time unless action is taken. Caries of the enamel may be arrested, or even recalcified, by plaque control regimes and fluoride application, provided that the basic enamel matrix structure is still intact. If cavitation of the enamel has however already occurred this may not be possible. For instance the concave surface of a small interproximal enamel lesion may not be reached by interdental flossing and in such a case a small repair by an adhesive filling material may be effective.

When the carious process reaches the dentine it is currently thought that a restoration of some sort must be made. If there is a number of large carious lesions of the dentine which cannot be restored within a short period of time, it is wise to prevent further increase in their size by temporarily dressing the teeth with a zinc oxide/eugenol cement. This process is know as stabilisation. Timely stabilisation may prevent pulpal damage and thus avoid the need for root canal therapy.

If stabilisation is to be fully effective, three simple criteria need to be satisfied:

- The cavity created should be retentive.
- The surrounding enamel should be strong enough to resist subsequent fracture.
- The enamel margins should be caries-free.

Such minimal preparation can be undertaken quickly for several teeth, often using only chisels and excavators and without resorting to rotary instruments. Sometimes this can be done without the need for local anaesthesia and if so, it may be possible to carry out stabilisation for teeth in several quadrants at one visit.

The carious lesion will be arrested by a combination of marginal seal, which prevents nutriment from reaching the causative bacteria, and by the antiseptic nature of the dressing material. Any pain attributable to dentine irritation will also be allayed. However, care should be taken with both history and examination to identify situations where the pain indicates severe and irreversible pulpitis or apical periodontitis. In such conditions a carious exposure may exist, implying an open pulpitis . If this were to be sealed by a stabilising dressing, severe pain and abscess formation could be precipitated due to the prevention of any means of drainage.

62 This ground section shows occlusally an extensive carious lesion of a size that would warrant stabilisation. The amount of both enamel and caries to be removed is indicated. Note that it is not necessary at this stage to make the preparation totally free of peripheral dentine caries. As such the preparation would not extend to sound or sensitive dentine so the need for local anaesthesia would be avoided.

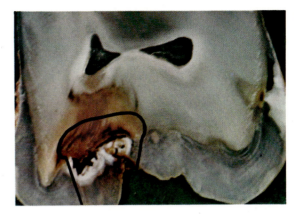

63 Large cavities in the lower molars have been stabilised with zinc oxide/eugenol dressings. Whilst still unset, their occlusal surfaces were contoured by the opposing teeth so that a traumatic occlusal relationship was avoided.

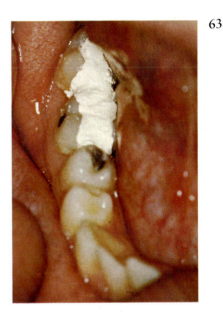

4 Pulp capping and partial pulpectomy

If the pulp of a tooth becomes exposed a choice has to be made from four possible treatment options:

Pulp capping
Partial pulpectomy
Pulpectomy
Extraction of the tooth

The first decision to be made is whether the interests of the patient are best served by saving the tooth. There should, of course, be no existent medical contra-indications. If it is decided to save the tooth then the best prognosis usually follows pulpectomy and complete root filling.

If however, successful pulpectomy is prejudiced by some complication such as an immature open apex or other anatomical difficulty, it may be necessary to resort to pulp capping or partial pulpectomy.

Pulp capping

The technique of pulp capping involves covering the exposure with a suitable dressing material in the expectation that the opening will be repaired by secondary dentine laid down by the pulp. Certain criteria however must be satisfied if this procedure is to be adopted with any hope of success:

- The pulp adjacent to the exposure should be vital and non-infected.
- The exposure should be small (<1.0 mm diameter).
- Blood should not exude in any quantity from the exposure.
- There should be no associated symptoms.
- The surrounding dentine should be sound and caries-free.

When all these criteria are satisfied there is a reasonable chance that repair will occur without any unfortunate sequelae. It may be difficult to assess accurately the absence of infection and the lack of symptoms does not always imply freedom from progressive pulpitis.

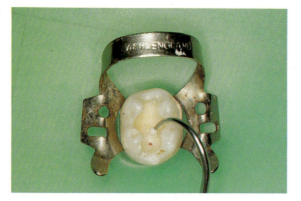

64–66 The pulp wound is first covered with a dressing, usually a quick setting proprietary calcium hydroxide material (**64**). This is to induce calcific repair and to sterilise any mild superficial contamination (Fisher, 1972). This may be introduced with a probe or calcium hydroxide applicator and allowed to flow over the wound without causing pressure on the pulp itself.

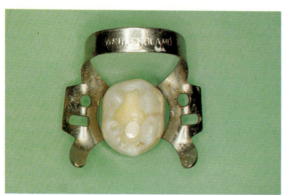

Two or three applications may be necessary (**65**) to build up a layer strong enough to withstand the placement of a base.

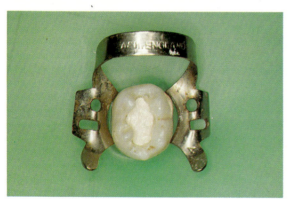

The base cement is placed in the usual way, care being taken not to dislodge or perforate the calcium hydroxide. The tooth is then ready to receive the permanent filling (**66**).

The tooth should be monitored over the next few months for any untoward symptoms. Should any occur then one of the other options will become necessary. If not, annual vitality tests and radiographs are undertaken to indicate whether the pulp has remained vital and whether a calcific barrier has been laid down.

Partial pulpectomy

Where the criteria for pulp capping cannot be satisfied and pulpectomy is contra-indicated, then partial pulpectomy may be considered as the only alternative to extraction. The criteria for this to be successful are that the tissue in the pulp canals, as opposed to the pulp chamber, should be deemed vital and free from infection.

Partial pulpectomy involves the removal of the coronal pulp tissue, leaving a clean small wound at the entrance to each pulp canal which can be dressed with a calcium hydroxide material in order to induce calcific repair.

A technique for partial pulpectomy has been described by Britton (1976). He states that a successful outcome is dependent on the tooth being vital, with no history of pain, and on the absence of excessive bleeding at the time of the pulpal excision which would suggest the absence of inflammation in the pulp canals. The younger the patient the better the prognosis.

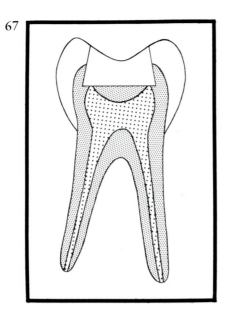

67

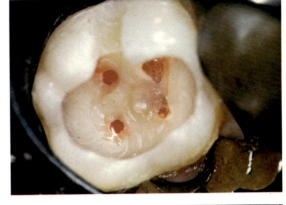

68

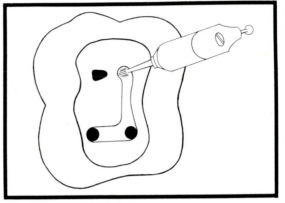

69

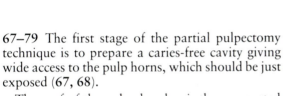

67–79 The first stage of the partial pulpectomy technique is to prepare a caries-free cavity giving wide access to the pulp horns, which should be just exposed (67, 68).

The roof of the pulp chamber is then separated from the tooth by a series of channels cut between the pulp horns (69, 70). Care should be taken to restrain the depth of cutting to the thickness of the dentine and to avoid unnecessary trauma to the pulp or introduction of debris into the pulp chamber.

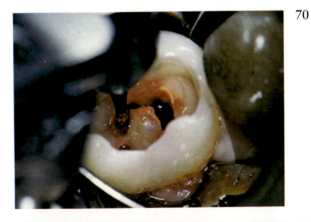

70

The roof of the pulp chamber can then be removed in one piece (71).

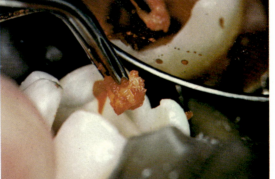

71

72

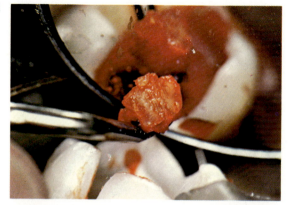

73

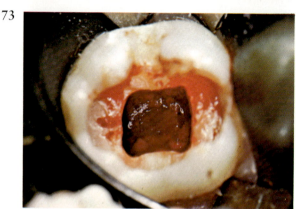

Amputation of the coronal portion of the pulp starts with its separation from the walls of the chamber by a large, sharp and sterile excavator. This excavator is then introduced between the pulp tissue and the chamber floor until it is in a position to sever the connection with the radicular pulp tissue. This should be done with a single clean cut across the entrance to each canal. The coronal pulp tissue can then be removed intact (**72, 73**). This will result in slight haemorrhage which can be absorbed by a small pledget of sterile cotton wool. If haemorrhage at this stage is excessive, this probably indicates an existing hyperaemia and so the prognosis for the satisfactory formation of a calcific barrier would be poor. Extraction of the tooth will therefore be the only viable treatment alternative.

74

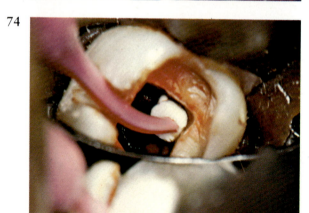

When haemorrhage has ceased, calcium hydroxide paste is introduced gently onto each pulp canal wound with the aid of a Jiffy tube (**74**). A small metal disc shaped from amalgam matrix band material is heat sterilised and placed onto the floor of the original cavity to create an artificial roof to the pulp chamber (**75**).

The metal disc, which has been cut considerably wider than the access to the pulp chamber, should be well supported by the cavity floor. It is held in place with zinc phosphate cement (**76**) and the remainder of the cavity is dressed with ZOE.

75

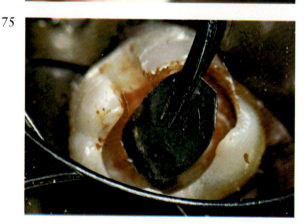

76

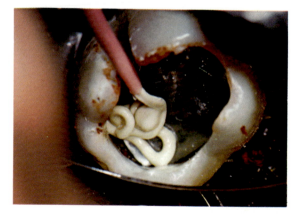

The completed partial pulpectomy is depicted in the line diagram 77 which shows the gap preserved between the wound dressing and the metal plate. This provides expansion space should it be required and thus prevents pressure being exerted on the healing pulp tissue. The advantage of this technique is that any heat from the tooth cutting is confined to the pulp chamber roof, well away from the radicular pulp. The secure metal plate protects this pulp tissue from pressure while the temporary cement is being compressed and so achieves sound marginal adaptation.

Successful healing will result in the formation of a calcific barrier over each pulp canal wound (78). The vitality of the tissue in each pulp canal and the integrity of each dentine bridge should be checked individually by re-opening the pulp chamber at approximately eight weeks post-operatively. After washing away the calcium hydroxide and blood clot the dentine bridges can be inspected (79) and an electric pulp test performed on each root in turn. Any canal that does not contain vital tissue should be root filled. The bridge areas are then re-dressed with calcium hydroxide and the tooth filled permanently with fortified zinc oxide/eugenol and amalgam.

Masterton (1966) has pointed out that the anatomy of the molar tooth is such that it allows a clean cut to be made when amputating the coronal pulp tissue. Because of this, haemorrhage is minimal and healing is by 'first intention' followed by dentine formation.

It is now generally recognised that partial pulpectomy on teeth with closed apices has a poor prognosis, often being followed by loss of vitality of any remaining pulp tissue. However, if immediate extraction is contra-indicated, this treatment may save the tooth for a few months, even years. It must be regarded as a treatment of last resort and the tooth should be monitored on a regular basis for any periapical bone changes.

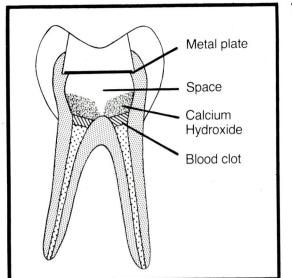

77

Metal plate

Space

Calcium Hydroxide

Blood clot

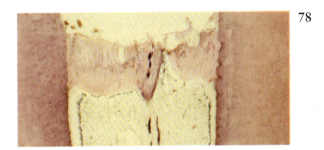

78

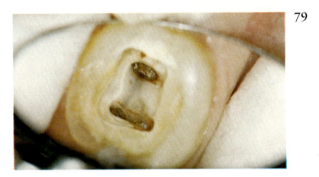

79

5 Suspicion of non-vitality

It is important during the examination of a patient to identify any tooth that is non-vital in order that appropriate treatment may be carried out as soon as possible. There is always the risk that an infected pulp may exacerbate into an acute periapical abscess if left untreated. Even if the condition remains chronic, changes in the periapical bone may progress considerably making eventual treatment more difficult than it need be. In patients with certain medical conditions, for instance valvular heart disease, a potential nidus of infection can be a serious health hazard. Thus a lookout should be kept for teeth which may be non-vital and where suspicion exists, tests for vitality should be made.

The following are some of the conditions under which a tooth may be suspected of being non-vital.

Tooth discolouration

80, 81 This extreme example (**80**), probably results from the pulp becoming hyperaemic following trauma. The discolouration is due to breakdown products from the excess of blood in the pulp, the pigments of which enter the dentinal tubules and are then visible through the translucent enamel. If there is no excess of blood in the pulp when it dies then the discolouration may be minimal (**81**).

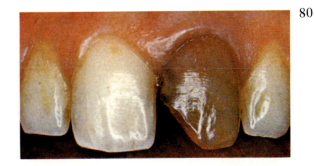
80

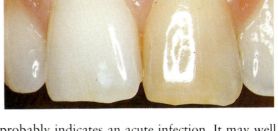
81

Signs of apical inflammation

82, 83 An abscess is about to point through the mucosa labially to the upper right central incisor (**82**). The source of this infection can be pulpal or periodontal. A negative pulp test response from the upper right central incisor will confirm the origin as being pulpal. The presence of a sinus or, less obviously, a small pinhead of scar tissue suggesting a healed sinus would be of equal significance. A more widespread reaction (**83**) than the chronic and well defined lesion of the previous figure probably indicates an acute infection. It may well be periodontal in origin and it is of diagnostic importance to perform vitality tests on all teeth in this region which might be involved, to eliminate the possibility of a pulpal cause.

82
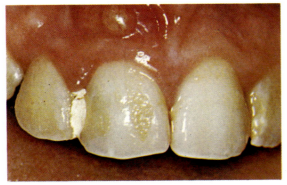

83
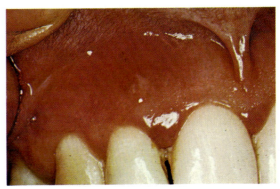

Excessively large restorations

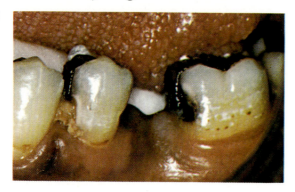

84 Any restoration (or carious lesion) which is considered large enough to have encroached on the pulp may well have caused pulp death. Here suspicion of the large restorations is greater due to the recurrent caries around the amalgams in the lower premolar and molar.

Fractured incisors

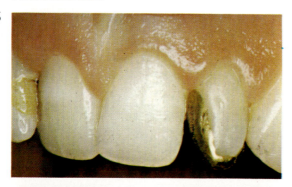

85 Fractured incisors are frequently found to be non-vital due the severing of apical blood vessels by the blow which fractured the crown. Other teeth may also have suffered such apical damage but without fracture to the crown. All teeth, upper or lower, which may have been affected by the blow must therefore be tested for vitality. Paradoxically, it is not unusual to find that the fractured tooth remains vital whilst adjacent unfractured teeth are discovered to be non-vital. If the injury occurred recently a negative response to vitality testing could merely indicate temporary concussion from which the pulp might recover. Such a tooth should be kept under regular review to allow possible recovery thereby obviating the need for root canal therapy.

Unlined silicate or composite restorations

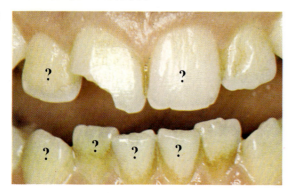

86, 87 Although this patient complained of tenderness of the upper left lateral incisor which was restored by a large gold inlay (**86**), routine vitality testing was performed on all the upper front six teeth. This confirmed that the upper left lateral was non-vital and further investigation showed that this had been caused by exposing the pulp during cavity preparation. However, the symptomless upper right lateral was also found to be non-vital though it had only a simple silicate or composite restoration. Radiographs revealed that the cavity floor was close to the pulp and a minute exposure may well have been created which led to death of the pulp and the extensive area of periapical bone loss (**87**). Unlined silicate fillings may also lead to pulp death even if the pulp is not exposed. This material is rarely used in modern dentistry but patients may be seen with longstanding silicate restorations dating from the pre-composite era.

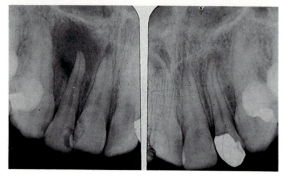

Other signs

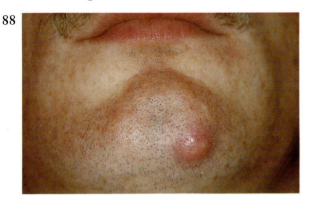

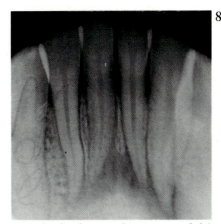

88, 89 Extra-oral signs may lead to the suspicion that a tooth may be non-vital. This mental abscess (**88**) was found to arise from the non-vital lower left incisor (**89**). Radiographically the periapical bone loss appears to involve both central incisors and the left lateral but positive vitality tests on the right central and left lateral incisors enabled the correct diagnosis to be made.

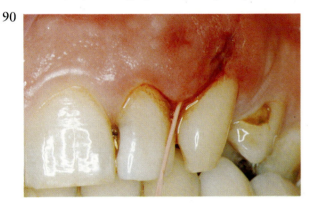

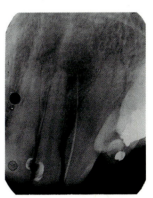

90, 91 An apical abscess can discharge down the periodontal ligament and into the gingival crevice (**90**) rather than through a labial sinus. Before taking a radiograph of the area it is helpful to insert a radiopaque marker, such as a gutta percha point, which will pass along the abscess track and identify the source of infection, in this case the upper left lateral incisor (**91**).

Testing for vitality

A tooth is considered to be vital if a response can be elicited from a stimulus applied to the dentine or through it to the pulp. If, therefore, a tooth's vitality is in doubt, the matter should either be resolved at examination stage or, if treatment is contemplated, it must be resolved before a local anaesthetic is administered. The simplest vitality procedure is, after briefing the patient, to start cavity preparation without anaesthesia. Sometimes, in cases of difficult diagnosis, cutting a small test cavity may be justified. If a sensitive response is elicited when dentine is reached this would indicate the presence of vital pulp tissue. A total lack of response would be strong evidence of non-vitality. Care must be taken in assuming normality when a positive response is obtained in a multi-rooted tooth. It is possible to have lost vitality in one root canal whilst maintaining it in another.

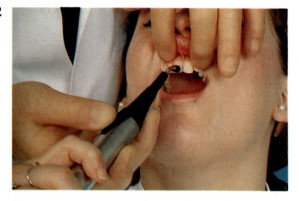

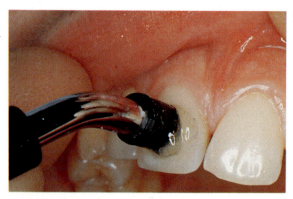

92, 93 Pulp testing is often performed using an electric pulp tester (EPT) of which there are many proprietary models available. The stimulus from such an instrument is capable of gradual variation which can be measured. However it is unwise to read too much significance into variations of response between teeth, even contralateral teeth, as there are many innocent factors which can affect this. The EPT is most useful in identifying a non-vital tooth by a zero response. False negatives are rare whereas false positives can occasionally cause confusion, particularly in multi-rooted teeth. One advantage of the EPT over other vitality tests is that a slow build up of stimulus is possible which ensures that the nervous patient cannot anticipate a positive response by confusing it with other stimuli such as pressure. Furthermore the level of response should be repeatable for any one tooth.

When the operator is wearing rubber gloves it is important, if false results are to be avoided, to obtain the necessary contact between the patient and the metal handle of the electric pulp tester by getting the patient to maintain finger contact with it throughout the test (**92**). Good electrical contact between the tester and the tooth is aided by a carbonised rubber tip and a gel (**93**). A tooth with a porcelain jacket crown presents obvious difficulties for electrical pulp testing due to the non-conductivity of the porcelain. If such a tooth is suspected of being non-vital and the matter cannot be resolved with the aid of a radiograph, it may be necessary to cut a small access hole through the cingulum area to the dentine. If the tooth proves vital this can be filled with composite with little harm having been done. If it proves to be non-vital then the access hole serves for the necessary root canal therapy.

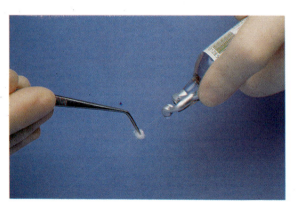

94, 95 A response to a cold stimulus can be a simple method of determining vitality and a particularly appropriate one if the symptom is of pain from cold. A small pledget of cotton wool is soaked in a highly volatile liquid such as ethyl chloride (**94**).

This can be applied to a dried tooth (95) to evoke a response to cold. Care must be taken to confine the pledget solely to the tooth under consideration. A negative response does not necessarily imply non-vitality. This is due to the fact that numerous factors could cause the pulp to be insulated from the cold stimulus. False positive results may occur from a periodontal response to pressure rather than a pulpal response to cold, particularly with the nervous patient.

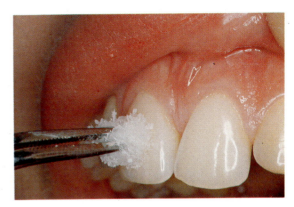

96 An alternative to cold is to apply a hot stimulus, useful in identifying which tooth is responsible for pain associated with hot food or drink. Gutta percha can be warmed and applied to the tooth. The tooth surface in this instance should be moist so that the gutta percha can be removed quickly if pain is caused. This method has drawbacks similar to those of ethyl chloride due to possible periodontal responses and the variability in temperature of the stimulus. A further disadvantage of the gutta percha technique is that heat applied to a gangrenous pulp can cause pain from the expansion of gases within the pulp which could be incorrectly interpreted as a normal vital response.

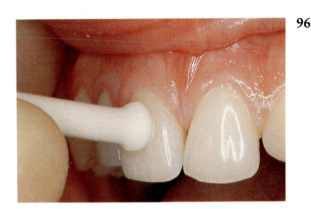

A simple positive response can often be obtained from touching dentine with a dental probe, should access to any be available. However not all such dentine is sensitive so that negative responses are of no value.

Root canal therapy

Whilst root canal therapy is an integral part of conservative dentistry its specialist nature makes monograph treatment more appropriate, e.g. Messing and Stock (1988).

6 Control of moisture and tissue retraction

Moisture in the mouth arises mainly from the saliva of the patient and the water introduced by the dentist for cooling or cleaning purposes. A minor source is from mucous glands, gingival haemorrhage and seepage of gingival fluid from the gingival crevice. Effective control of this moisture is essential for a variety of reasons.

Patient comfort

The patient cannot remain comfortable and relaxed whilst fluid is collecting in the mouth. This can be particularly distressing for the patient in the supine position. There is a risk that this might give rise to swallowing at a time when closing the mouth could be dangerous, for instance, during cavity preparation.

Operating efficiency

To avoid delays due to the patient wishing to empty his mouth at frequent intervals.

Visibility

The fine detail of much in restorative dentistry can only be seen when the tooth concerned is dry. During cavity preparation, however, a water spray is required to avoid overheating the dentine and pulp. At this time one of the most difficult things to achieve is good visibility.

Avoidance of contamination

Unless adequately controlled, fluids can act as a separating medium between the tooth substance and dental material being applied i.e. lining, base, fissure sealant, acid-etched composite or cement and so prevent proper adherence. The physical properties of many filling materials will deteriorate if moisture contamination is allowed to occur. Delayed expansion will follow moisture contamination of zinc containing amalgams for instance. Impression materials will fail to record detail accurately if the surfaces concerned are not dry. This is particularly so with silicone based impression materials which are repellent to water.

Control of sepsis

Saliva, being highly infected, must be prevented from entering the pulp chamber during root canal therapy when sterility is to be achieved.

Methods of moisture control

The problems set by these requirements of fluid control can be solved by the use of one or more of the following:

- Suction – high volume
          – low volume
- Air jet
- Absorbent material
- Isolation
- Styptics and coagulants

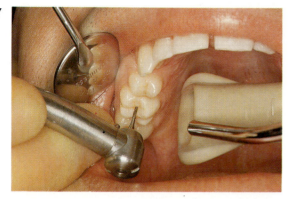

97 During cavity preparation, the water coolant can be removed from the mouth by a high volume aspirator operated by a chairside assistant. If the apparatus is efficient and the working end properly placed, all the water, together with tooth and filling debris, will be removed before it can fall to the back of the mouth, thus making other devices unnecessary.

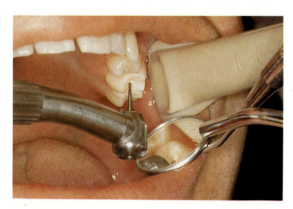

98 The chairside assistant can also aid visibility by retracting soft tissues, in this case the cheek, with the aspirator nozzle and by keeping the mirror clear of water droplets with a continuous stream of air from the air syringe.

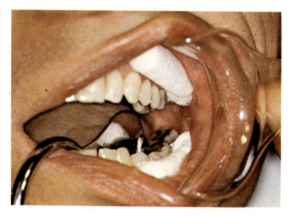

99 Prior to the insertion of filling materials, dryness of the teeth is obtained with an air jet and maintained most simply by the combined use of cotton wool rolls and saliva ejector. These are the absolute minimum requirements of moisture control if restorative work of a high standard is to be achieved.

The cotton wool rolls are placed in the buccal sulci to absorb salivary secretions from the parotid duct and from the mucous glands in the cheek. If lower teeth are being treated the saliva ejector should possess a tongue flange to keep the tongue away from the site of operation. This can sometimes be aided with a further cotton wool roll placed between the ejector flange and the teeth. The saliva ejector will remove secretions from the sub-maxillary and sub-lingual glands and, with the patient's assistance, will keep the floor of the mouth from lifting and spilling saliva into the tooth.

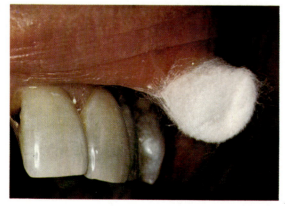

100 Care should be exercised in removing cotton wool rolls especially if they have been in place for some time in a fairly dry mouth. This is because the roll may have become adherent to the mucosa and if removed forcibly, can tear the soft tissue. Here it can be seen that the roll is well attached to the lip and will need to be sprayed with water to release it without causing damage.

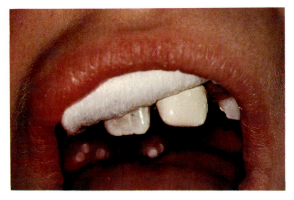

101

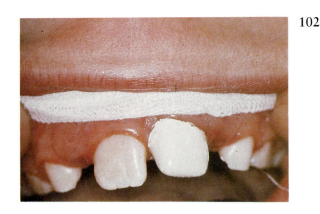

102

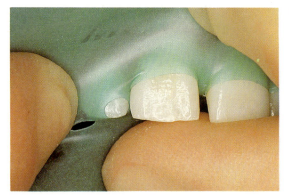

103

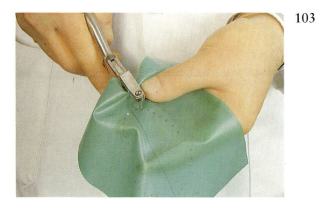

104

101, 102 Sometimes, particularly in young patients and patients with short upper lips, there is not room to place a roll so that it does not obscure vision and access (**101**). In this eventuality a small roll of dental gauze can be substituted. The less bulky gauze can be placed out of sight in the sulcus. In this view (**102**) the lip has been lifted to show it.

103–108 To obtain a perfectly dry and sterile field, protected even from the moisture of the patient's exhaled air, a rubber dam should be used. Pre-cut sheets of strong rubber are now available with a high resistance to tearing.

A series of appropriately spaced holes is punched in a sheet of rubber (**103**). The dam is passed between the teeth by 'knifing' one edge of each interdental piece of rubber past the contact point (**104**). This can be facilitated by lubricating the dam with a light grease.

When the clinical crown is fully through the dam the margin is inverted by the use of a plastic instrument, aided by an air stream (**105**). This is done to get the dam as far as possible from the operating field and to achieve the best possible gingival seal.

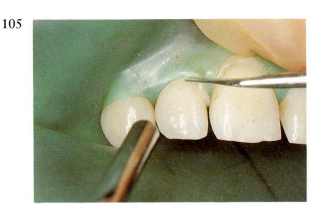

105

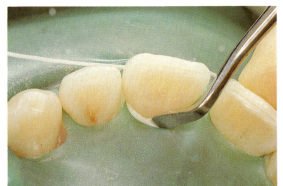

106

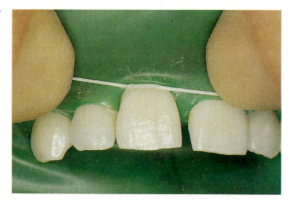

107

For good retention round anterior teeth it is advisable to involve two teeth on either side of the one to be treated. Retention is further assisted with ligatures of dental floss which are pushed past the cingulum palatally and onto the taper of the root (**106**) and then tied with the double 'surgeon's' knot (**107**). This will prevent the rubber dam from slipping towards the incisal margin and will keep it in the gingival crevice.

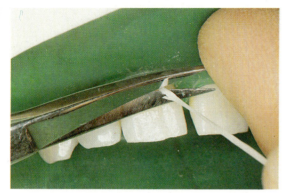

108

The loose ends should always be cut close to the knot (**108**) to keep them out of the field of operation. Sterility is then achieved when necessary by swabbing both tooth and dam with a suitable antiseptic.

109 If there is the risk of the rubber dam being displaced by pressure from the patient's lips and cheeks, the distal ends of the dam may be held firmly in place with rubber dam clamps. Here a premolar clamp has been applied to the first premolar and it will be noted that it has not been necessary to put this tooth through the dam.

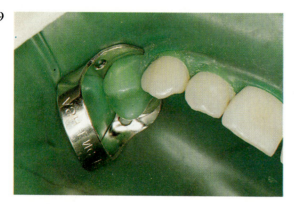

109

110, 111 An alternative to the clamp, provided that tight contact points exist, is to use a thin strip of rubber which can be stretched (**110**) and then wedged between two teeth (**111**).

When applied, the perimeter of the dam needs to be held back with a frame to prevent it obstructing the operator's view or access to the teeth.

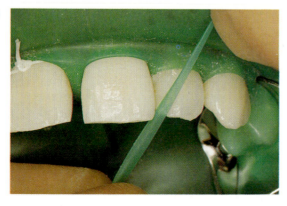

110

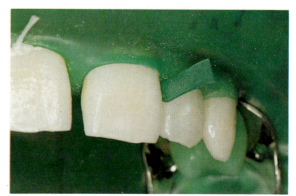

111

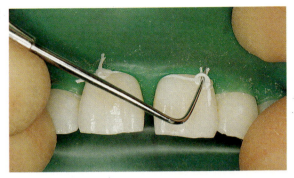

112

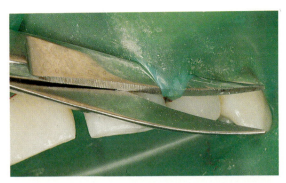

113

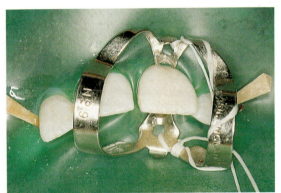

114

112, 113 To remove the dam the ligatures are first taken off, the knots being picked undone with the aid of a dental probe (**112**). Removal of the dam itself is facilitated by stretching labially each interdental section in turn to allow it to be cut with scissors (**113**).

114 The so-called 'butterfly' clamp can be used on incisor teeth if the ligatures prove difficult to apply or retain, as on teeth without a pronounced cingulum. However such a clamp does restrict access, particularly if a matrix strip has to be used for a filling. The clamp may also be superimposed on a radiograph and obscure some important detail in root canal therapy.

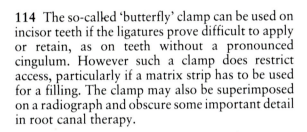

115

115 Many operators now use rubber dam for most of their restorative work. The upper first molar here has been well isolated for filling with amalgam. It is claimed that much time can be saved and patient comfort provided by the application of rubber dam before cavity preparation is started.

For posterior teeth it is considered by some operators to be an advantage to use wingless clamps which can be placed on the tooth prior to dam placement. The dam, suitably lubricated, can then be slipped into place over the clamp. This technique allows much better vision for the application of the clamp. There is therefore less likelihood of gingival trauma than when the dam is fixed to a winged clamp before it is inserted in the mouth.

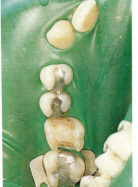

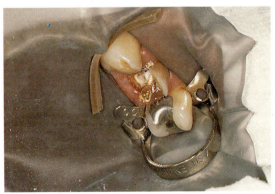

116

116 It is not always possible to apply the rubber to a particular tooth, perhaps because it is broken down to gum level or because it is a bridge abutment. In such cases a split dam technique can be used whereby the dam is cut to allow the teeth on either side of the one in question through the same hole in the dam. This does not give total isolation but it can still be a great aid to moisture control and will protect the airway.

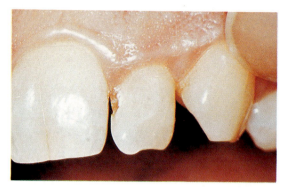

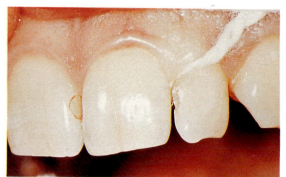

117, 118 A local papillitis (**117**) may make access for cavity preparation difficult and consequent gingival haemorrhage and seepage may contaminate the restoration during insertion if rubber dam is applied. Retraction of the papilla and a dry field may be obtained by the insertion of a length of adrenalin impregnated cord (**118**). The gingival blanching seen here indicates the effect of pressure from the string, which has produced a local ischaemia. Haemostasis will be further assisted by the adrenalin.

119 The creation of a dry gingival crevice, immediately prior to taking impressions of a subgingival preparation, can be greatly assisted by the use of an alum/adrenalin solution (Wilson and Tay, 1977). A drop of this solution (Appendix 3) is picked up between the beaks of the tweezers (arrowed) and introduced into the gingival crevice. After a minute the crevice is washed and dried. The adrenalin acts as a haemostatic and the alum causes

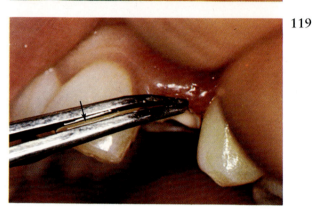

precipitation of gingival fluid, thus providing a dry field. The technique is also of value in obtaining dryness in the gingival region during the packing of amalgam cavities. Because of the possibility of absorption of adrenalin through the gum this solution should not be used on patients for whom adrenalin is contra-indicated.

Protection of the airway

During dental treatment it is important to ensure that foreign bodies do not pass via the pharynx into the gut or the trachea and lungs. The risk is particularly high when the patient is supine and items dropped into the mouth can fall directly into the pharnyx if this is not effectively sealed at the time by contact between the soft palate and the tongue.

The variety of such foreign bodies is considerable, including pieces of tooth or filling, burs, calculus, dentine pins, reamers and files, root filling points, crowns, bridges or inlays. The ideal protection is provided by rubber dam but this is not always practicable.

120

120 A 'butterfly' sponge, with a safety cord attached, may be used to protect the pharynx whenever there is the risk of a foreign body falling to the back of the mouth. This should be softened by moistening with water and placed half in the mouth and half outside as illustrated.

7 Bases and varnishes

Bases and varnishes are materials placed in cavities, for a variety of reasons, before the final fillings or restorations are inserted (Appendix 4). Which material to use will vary with the size and depth of the cavity and the filling material to be inserted.

121 The classical amalgam cavity cut just into dentine only requires a varnish before the insertion of the amalgam. This helps to prevent marginal percolation prior to the formation of corrosion products which will eventually fulfil the same function. If a base were to be included the cavity would become too shallow and the resulting amalgam restoration would be weakened. Further deepening of the cavity solely to make room for a base is unwarranted. (N.B. This illustration shows unacceptable damage to the adjacent tooth which should have been avoided by a more careful technique (see **151**) or by protection with a metal matrix band.)

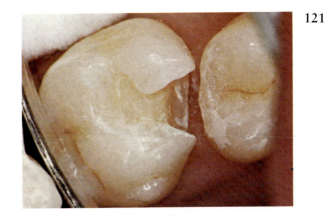
121

122–125 The deep cavity, where the caries is deemed to have approached closely to the pulp (**122**) needs to be lined. This is done in three stages for an amalgam restoration.

First a wash of calcium hydroxide is placed on the pulpal floor (**123**). Then the depth of the cavity is reduced to classical proportions with a structural base (**124**). Finally the cavity walls and floor are given a coat of varnish.

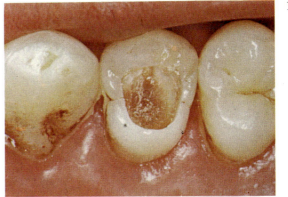
122

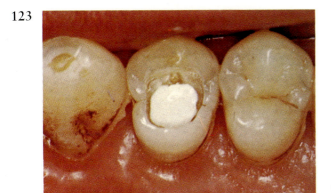
123

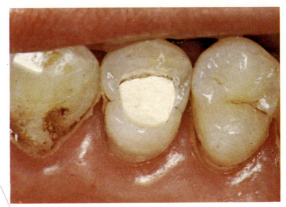
124

125

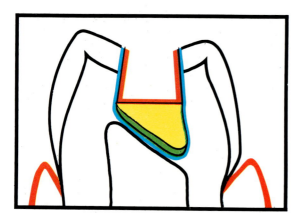

All three stages can be summarised in diagrammatic form (125).

126

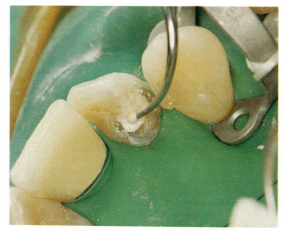

126 Protection from irritation of the dentine is recommended beneath a composite restoration. This can be achieved most readily with a quick setting calcium hydroxide cement introduced with an applicator or small brush. It is advisable to use an acid resistant type of cement in order to reduce the likelihood of dissolution of the calcium hydroxide during the acid-etching stage.

In this view a ball-ended applicator has placed a drop of calcium hydroxide cement on the axial floor of the cavity and is spreading this to cover all the exposed dentine. Eugenol containing cements should be avoided due to the deleterious effect of the eugenol on the composite filling material.

127

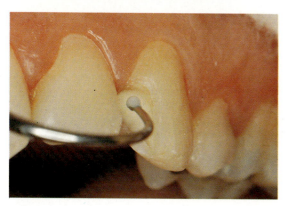

128

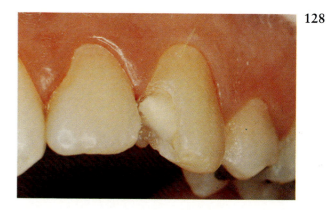

127–130 The relative blandness of glass ionomer (polyalkenoate) cement to the pulp allows its frequent use as a base material. Nevertheless in deep cavities a sub-base of a calcium hydroxide containing cement is advisable. The glass ionomer has the added advantage over calcium hydroxide of being adhesive to dentine. This, and its naturally rough surface improves the retention of large composite fillings by micro-mechanical means. The glass ionomer is applied similarly with a ball-ended applicator (127) and should cover all available dentine (128).

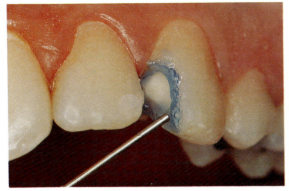

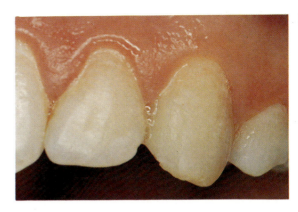

The enamel walls are etched (129) if composite is to be the filling material (130). It is not necessary to etch the glass ionomer surface as it has been shown (Taggert and Pearson, 1988) that composite adheres very well to it without this procedure. Rubber dam should be used unless total moisture control can be guaranteed throughout the insertion of this type of restoration.

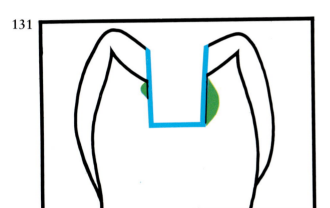

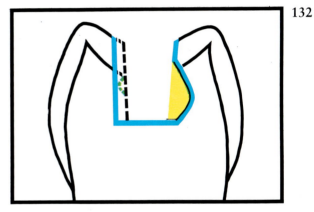

131, 132 Minimal depth gold inlay cavities require no base. A certain amount of thermal insulation is provided by the cement with which an inlay is retained. A cement may however be required to reduce the depth of a very deep cavity or to eradicate undercuts.

Minor undercuts (131, left) should be removed during cavity preparation (132, left). Where however an undercut is considerable, due to the extensive spread of caries at the amelo-dentinal junction (131, right), a choice has to be made between cutting back or blocking out. To cut back the overlying enamel may so weaken the cusp that it has to be capped (see 313) and it may be preferable to achieve withdrawal form by eliminating the undercut with cement (132, right).

8 Modern approach to minimum carious lesions

Since the ninetenth century Black's principles of cavity preparation, perhaps with minor modifications, have applied in dentistry. They still apply for carious lesions of 'classical' proportions and for traditional restorations which may be in need of replacement.

In the case of minimal carious lesions, however, one principle in particular - that of extension for prevention - is challenged for its relevance to modern dentistry. This principle demanded the inclusion in the cavity outline of any sites of adjacent tooth which might conceivably become carious in the future, for instance all occlusal fissures and any interproximal enamel surfaces that could not be reached by the toothbrush bristle.

Adoption of this principle will result in the loss of much sound tooth tissue thus greatly weakening the tissue which remains. Any restoration has only a limited life-span and will need replacing several times during the life of the patient. As Elderton (1990) has pointed out each replacement will inevitably remove more sound tissue thus adding to the problem. The modern view is that such loss of sound tissue is frequently unnecessary and is therefore unjustified.

In many countries the advent of fluoride in water supplies and toothpastes has resulted in the slowing down of the carious process. Preventive techniques in general use can arrest and even reverse the advance of a lesion or prevent the development of recurrent caries in previously vulnerable sites.

It is now considered that where the patient can be expected to use a toothbrush with a fluoride toothpaste regularly and apply dental floss wherever practicable, recurrent caries can be kept at bay. The outline form of any cavity, where these conditions pertain, should now be determined solely by the extent of the present carious lesion rather than its possible future progress. Such a philosophy should reduce considerably the occurrence, in later life, of fractured cusps and the need for extensive and expensive restorations.

It will be apparent therefore that there is no such thing as the 'classical' cavity for minimal lesions. The operator will not be able to proceed with his textbook vision of the stereotype cavity; he will need to think as he goes along and modify his cavity form in the light of what he discovers on the way.

Another of Black's principles, that of retention form, requires modification as a consequence of the choice of filling material. If an adhesive material is appropriate then the unnecessary removal of tooth tissue to provide mechanical retention, in the form of undercuts, can be avoided.

In some situations these considerations can lead to the use of a combination of filling materials, for instance amalgam and composite, in the same restoration.

Perhaps the most dramatic change to be observed from the application of this approach is in the treatment of the Class II lesion with minimal dentine involvement but without evidence of occlusal fissure caries. Adherence to Black's principles would result in a wide interproximal box, visible both buccally and lingually, with an occlusal keyway and lock involving all occlusal fissures (see 121). Adoption of a modern approach, for the same lesion, would result in a self-retentive box with virtually no occlusal involvement and seen only in the marginal ridge region as a narrow filling (see 159).

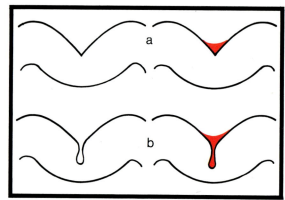

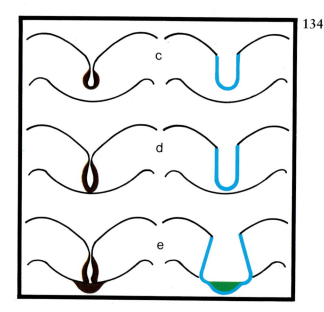

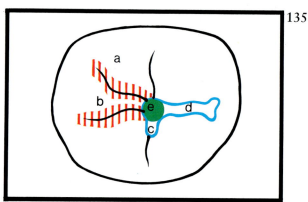

Occlusal fissures

133 An occlusal fissure may be caries-free and exists in one of two forms: as a surface wrinkle with little depth, (a); or as a lack of fusion between cusps of enamel which extends part way, (b); or even totally through the enamel thickness.

Such fissures do not require any attention in the clean mouth with a low or nonexistent caries rate. If plaque control is doubtful then it may be advisable to seal them with a resin fissure sealant (magenta - right).

It is not usually possible to distinguish these two fissures by simple observation of the occlusal surface and they should not be probed to find out as this might create ideal conditions for the initiation of caries. Neither should they be included in the outline of any cavity being cut in their vicinity though they may benefit from sealing as an adjunct to the adjacent filling in a procedure now known as a preventive resin restoration.

134 Problems can exist for the diagnosis of caries in discoloured fissures and again the temptation to resort to the probe should be resisted. Bitewing radiographs may help by revealing caries of the dentine at the amelo-dentinal junction but the guiding rule should be if in doubt wait, or fissure seal.

If no doubt exists and cavity preparation of part of the occlusal surface is embarked upon, there will be an ideal opportunity to observe a cross-sectional view of all the fissures. It will then be possible to determine whether or not they are carious and to take appropriate action. Each fissure should be assessed individually as cavity preparation continues.

Caries of a fissure (brown), if seen from within the cavity, will extend to one of three levels, part way through the enamel, (c); totally through the

enamel but not involving dentine, (d); or extending into dentine, (e). Each of these levels is treated on its merits by only cutting out the fissure to the depth of the carious involvement (blue). Where only enamel is involved (c & d, right) an acid-etched composite restoration should be placed as it is inappropriate and impracticable to fill the cavity with amalgam. The part of the cavity involved with caries of the dentine (e, left) can be dealt with on more traditional lines (e, right), if amalgam is preferred, by an undercut cavity (blue) and a base of lining material (green).

135 This diagram of a seemingly odd cavity combines all the five approaches to occlusal fissures shown in **133** and **134**, fissure sealing (a & b); fissure filling (c & d); and amalgam filling (e). Any or all of these may be required for the same tooth.

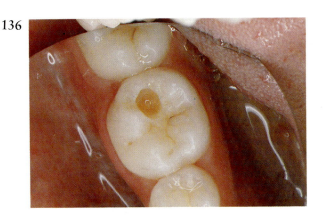

136

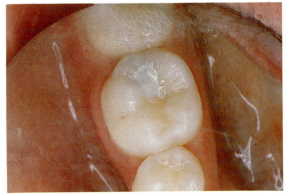

137

136, 137 A clinical example using Ketac Silver (Espe, GmbH, D-8031, Seefeld/Oberbay) demon-strates the result of treating fissures only where required.

Interproximal carious lesions

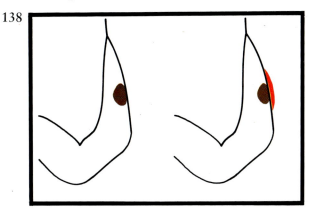

138

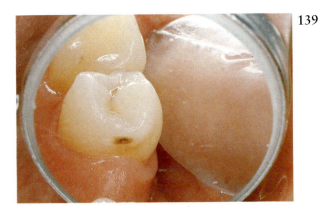

139

138, 139 Signs of early caries, such as an enamel white spot without signs of cavitation (**138** left), can often be seen interproximally on posterior teeth. This may be possible because the adjacent tooth is either missing (**139**) or being prepared for a Class II restoration at the time. The opportunity should be taken to clean and etch the lesion and to cover it with unfilled resin (magenta - **138**, right) or coat it with a fluoride varnish e.g. Duraphat. This would prevent the progression of the lesion the treatment of which, at a later date, would involve access being gained through the marginal ridge.

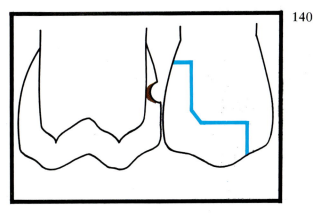

140

140–143 If cavitation has already occurred without dentine involvement (**140**, brown) then something more than a resin coating will be required.

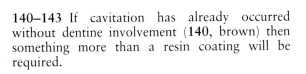

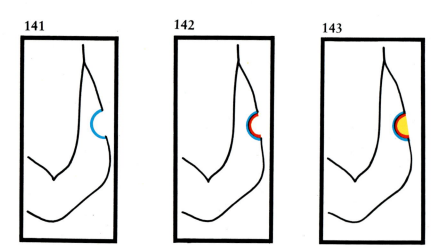

Saucerisation with a round bur will remove the carious enamel and freshen up the perimeter of sound enamel (141 - blue). This can then be etched and coated with resin (142 - magenta) before filling with composite (143, yellow).

144–159 When interproximal caries involving dentine is diagnosed (144, 145) and direct access is not possible then access for treating the lesion has to be obtained through the marginal ridge, or less frequently via the occlusal or buccal surface in the so-called tunnel preparation approach. If the fissures of the occlusal surface are sound then they will not be involved in the preparation and so a cavity consisting of a self-retentive box should be the preparation of choice.

An access hole is cut with a small-diameter, round-ended fissure bur starting just inside the marginal ridge (146) and progressing to a position slightly cervical to the caries (147).

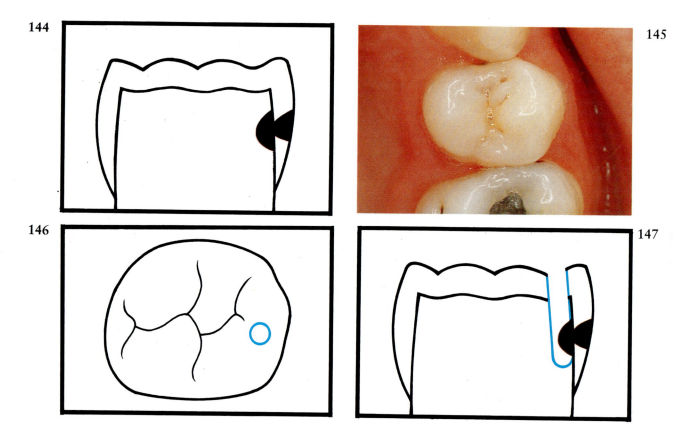

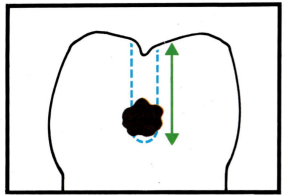

148

149

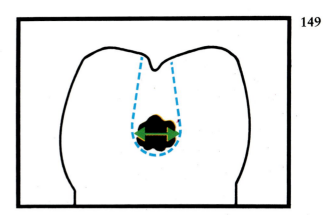

This is also demonstrated in figure **148** where it will be noticed that the caries buccal and lingual to the access hole has not been eliminated. This can be removed by slight tilting of the bur buccally and lingually (**149** arrowed). Seen from above the access hole (**150** - blue) remains minimal, the divergence of the box walls being denoted by broken blue lines.

150

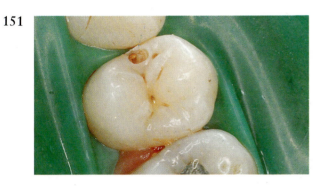

151

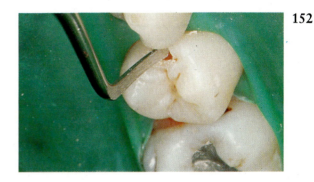

152

So far the adjacent tooth has been protected from damage by preservation of the interproximal enamel (**151**). This can be removed safely by the use of narrow chisels (**152**) and cervical margin trimmers. The enamel of the box walls can be strengthened into butt joints (**153, 154**).

153

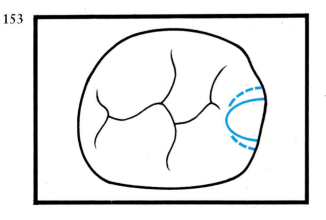

154

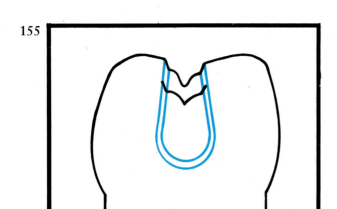

The interproximal view (155) demonstrates how this cavity has been restrained to the minimum size required for access and removal of caries. The rounded end of the bur has produced a pear shaped outline, avoiding unwelcome sharp line-angles, which is easier to pack.

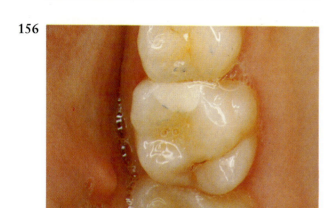

If an adhesive restorative filling material is to be used, the cavity is now complete and the tooth can be filled with composite (156) or glass ionomer.

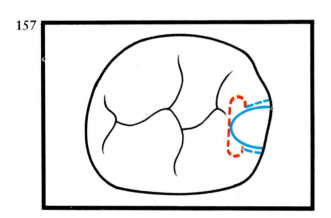

For amalgam however some substitute is required for the absent classical keyway and lock if full retention form is to be achieved. This is introduced with a very small round bur which can cut grooves carefully confined to the dentine (157 and 158 - magenta). The final restoration (159) is seen to be no bigger than the size required to gain access and deal with the caries.

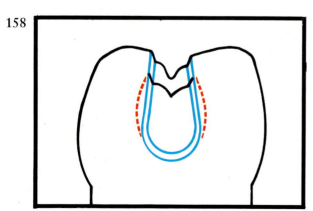

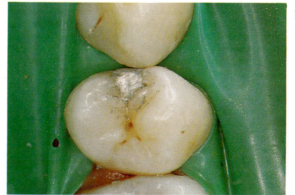

The tunnel preparation

160–165 Where occlusal and interproximal caries are separated by a sound marginal ridge it may be possible to preserve the ridge by adopting the tunnel preparation. Obvious recurrent occlusal caries can be seen in the most distal of the fissures of the upper first molar (160) and when this is dealt with, the inner aspects of an interproximal lesion are revealed (161). With care, and helped by tooth separation effected by means of a wedge, the caries can be removed without damage to the adjacent tooth (162). On close inspection the green of the rubber dam can be seen outlining the finished cervical margin of the cavity.

Difficulty of access for the manipulation of enamel finishing instruments makes it impossible to trim unsupported enamel from the interproximal margins and thus amalgam is an inappropriate material for use here. However Ketac Silver, an adhesive restorative material, will give support to the marginal enamel. Being a sintered mixture of the ceramic glass ionomer and metallic silver, it is known as a cermet material, (McLean and Gasser, 1985). It is introduced from the nozzle of the Ketac capsule after inserting a metal matrix strip interproximally (163). This will limit any excess (164) which can be removed with carving instruments and polishing strips (165).

Ketac Silver can be used as the sole filling material but, if greater strength is required to resist occlusal stresses, the occlusal portion of the cavity may be filled with amalgam.

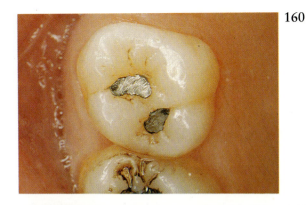

160

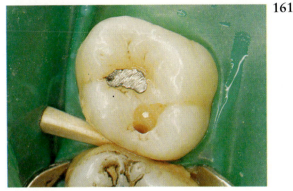

161

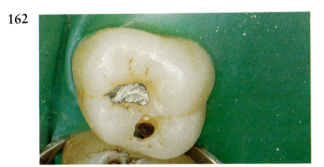

162

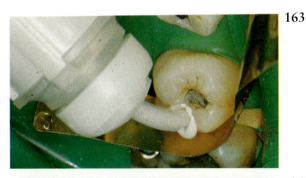

163

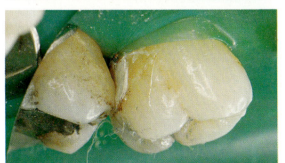

164

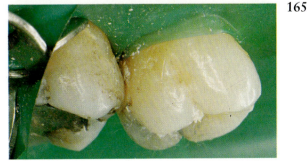

165

166

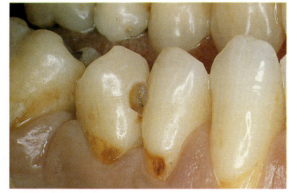

166 It is sometimes possible to deal with interproximal caries through a tunnel from the buccal surface thus preserving the occlusal surface totally intact.

Posterior composite restorations

Composite resin has not yet been totally accepted into dentistry for all types of posterior restoration. There is the problem of polymerisation shrinkage, particularly in large direct restorations. Attempts are being made to overcome this with the use of indirect composite inlays. Another difficulty can arise in Class II restorations which extend cervically past the amelo-cemental junction. Here the lack of enamel precludes the acid-etch technique from being effective at the cervical margin thus risking possible marginal leakage (Shortall *et al.*, 1989). These objections do not apply to the minimal Class I restoration and here composite can be the ideal restorative material to use in the type of cavity shown in **135**.

167

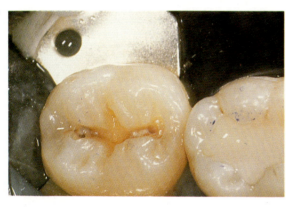

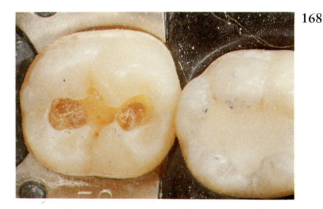

168

167–171 In this molar (**167**) the fissures have been run out as described in diagram **134** (middle) revealing caries of the dentine below the mesial and distal fissures. This is dealt with (**168**) along the lines indicated in **134** (bottom).

The areas of dentine involvement are lined with a calcium hydroxide cement (**169**) and after etching of the enamel margins (**170**) the cavity is filled with composite (**171**). Any untouched fissures may be sealed with unfilled resin.

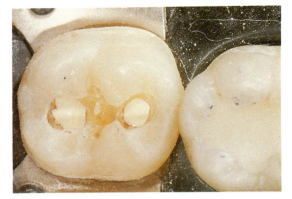
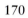

169

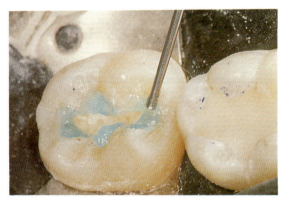

170

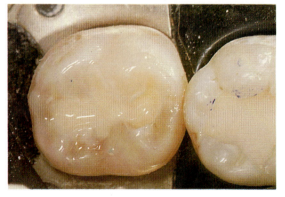

171

9 Traditional amalgam restorations

172 There is still the need to understand and to undertake Black's traditional or modified cavity preparations. This may be either because a carious lesion has not been identified for treatment before it has reached a considerable size, or because for some time to come, there will be many existing traditional restorations that will need replacement due to development of secondary caries.

Most textbooks of Restorative and Operative Dentistry deal at length with all aspects of such amalgam restorations. It is not intended therefore to cover exhaustively such a large subject in this book. A number of examples have been selected of points particularly worth visual emphasis

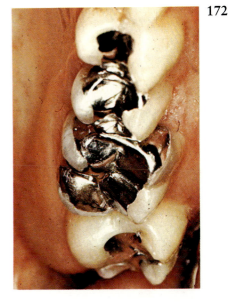

172

Cavity preparation

173 For reasons both of pulpal integrity and for maximum preservation of sound tooth tissue, the depth of the cavity should be cut, in the first instance, just into dentine, giving a cavity depth of about 2.5mm. When the outline form has been established and all peripheral caries eliminated, any remaining pulpal caries is then removed by the careful use of a large sharp excavator directed so as to avoid direct pressure towards the pulp. This is a fail-safe procedure as sound dentine will not be removed thus avoiding a traumatic exposure. A bur, which is by design capable of removing both carious and non-carious dentine, carries this risk. Some operators recommend a bur for removal of pupal caries but they are always careful to qualify how it should be used - a large, round slow speed bur revolving slowly in a conventional handpiece.

The resultant cavity form is shown in blue. It is dangerous to cut a flat floor at the maximum depth of the caries as there would be a risk of causing a pulpal exposure. Furthermore, it will unnecessarily remove sound dentine (as shown in red).

174 The cervical margin of a Class II cavity should, wherever possible, be kept slightly supra-gingival. Several benefits will accrue from this. Gingival trauma during cavity preparation

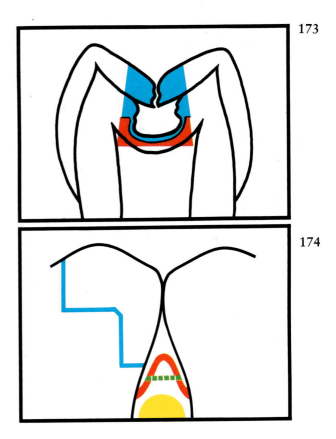

173

174

and matrix placement should not occur, thus eliminating problems of gingival haemorrhage which might contaminate the base and amalgam during insertion. In addition the cervical margin of the restoration will be readily accessible to the patient to aid plaque control and periodontal irritation from a plaque retentive sub-gingival margin will be avoided.

Extensive caries, however, often extends sub-gingivally and may be the cause of a periodontal pocket. In such instances, a supra-gingival relationship can be obtained for the restoration margin by the removal of gingival tissue as indicated by the green line. This can most readily be undertaken by surgical diathermy (see **295**).

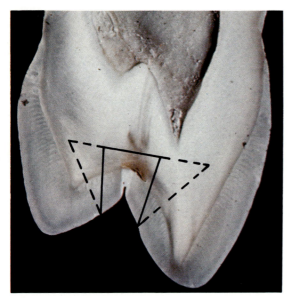

175

175, 176 Ideally the cavo-surface angle around an amalgam restoration should be 90⁰. This is to provide a sound butt-joint between amalgam and enamel.

In teeth with steep cusps, as in this upper first premolar (**175**), creation of a 90⁰ cavo-surface angle (broken line) would result in an excessively wide cavity floor and considerable weakening of the cusps. This is avoided by cutting as indicated by the solid line. In order to achieve a strong 90⁰ margin in the finished amalgam restoration, it should be carved as depicted in **176** and if necessary, the opposing cusp should be reduced to make room for the restoration. Any attempt to reproduce the original occlusal contour (**176**, lower broken line) would result in a weak margin to the restoration.

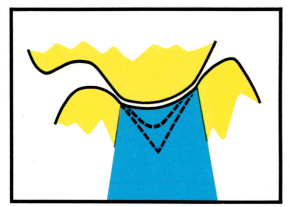

176

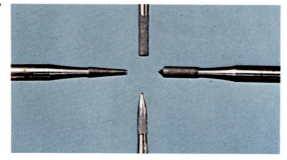

177

177 Diamond and tungsten carbide cutting burs can leave cavity margins rough and irregular (Boyde *et al.*, 1972) and these require smoothing with finishing burs. The finishing burs depicted here have distinct advantages for doing this over more traditional finishing burs. They are used in the turbine handpiece, the high speed of which allows very smooth application to the enamel without snatching or running out of the cavity. Being without blades they smooth the margins without dislodging enamel prisms (Baker and Curson, 1974). They cut by virtue of longitudinal scratches which get eliminated with use. These can be replaced and the burs 'resharpened' by scoring lengthways with a hand held diamond bur.

Minimally extended box walls may not allow access to a finishing bur and these margins may be smoothed with chisels and cervical margin trimmers.

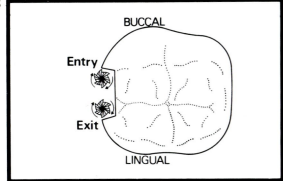

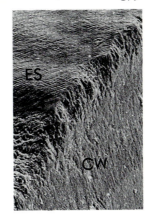

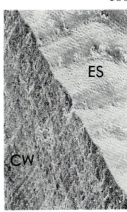

178–180 Boyde has drawn attention to the effect of the direction of bur rotation on the quality of the enamel margin produced on the box walls of a Class II cavity. This is related to whether the bur blades are rotating into the cavity, an 'entry' cut, or out of the cavity, an 'exit' cut. Tronstad and Leidal (1974) have illustrated this diagrammatically (178) and shown with the SEM that with an 'exit' bur rotation, enamel is torn out of the cavity leaving a very rough margin (179) whereas with an 'entry' rotation the margin is left intact (180). Where the direction of rotation for a bur can be altered, an 'entry' rotation should be chosen for finishing enamel margins. Where this is not possible a rough margin must be expected and this can be smoothed as indicated above (177).

Packing, carving and polishing the Class II amalgam restoration

181–188 A Class II cavity requires a matrix band to support the amalgam during condensation. When in place, this should be contoured with a ball-ended burnisher to mimic the original convex tooth shape. This is especially important when making contact between the matrix band and the adjacent tooth. The band should also be tightly wedged at its cervical margin to prevent the extrusion of excess amalgam. Packing of the amalgam should start in the deepest part of the box and extend into the corners, (181).

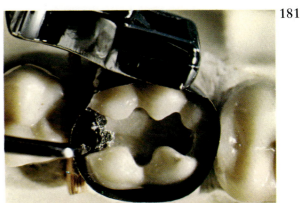

181

Good adaptation without porosity is achieved through firm hand pressure with small pluggers of appropriate cross-sectional shape. To adapt into the line angles of the box this shape should be rhomboidal or lozenge. Condensation in the later stages is obtained using larger diameter pluggers and may be aided by mechanical vibration. This can make the process of condensation less tiring. It should continue until there is a considerable excess of amalgam (182).

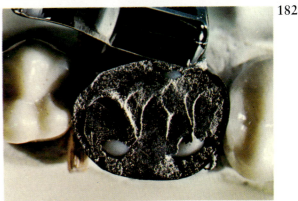

182

183

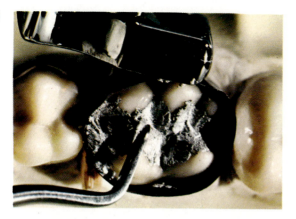

The gross excess is then removed and the accessible portions roughly carved before the matrix band is removed (**183**). This carving is particularly critical in the marginal ridge area if the ridge is not to fracture unfavourably when the matrix band is removed. Support can be given to the marginal ridge with a plugger at this critical time.

184

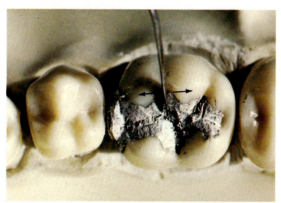

Carving is completed with a sharp hand instrument such as a Ward's (**184**) or Hollenback carver. Occlusally this should be worked parallel to the cavity margin (arrowed) with the blade held partly on the cusp slope whilst cutting the amalgam. In this way the cusp slopes act as a template to reproduce the natural shape in the amalgam and to prevent the formation of negative margins. Thin articulating paper, such as GHM (see **501**) can be used to detect any high spots or premature contacts which should be removed before dismissing the patient.

185

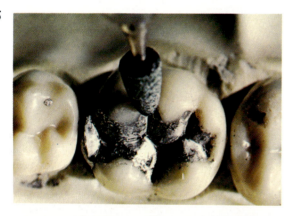

Finishing and polishing cannot be started until a future visit when the amalgam will have set hard. Any sizeable reduction may be undertaken with a carborundum point (**185**). The use of this should however be kept to a minimum as it deeply scores the surface. Final shaping is achieved with a finishing bur (**186**).

186

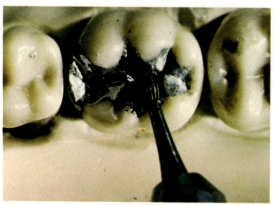

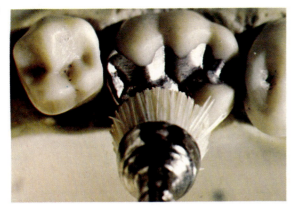

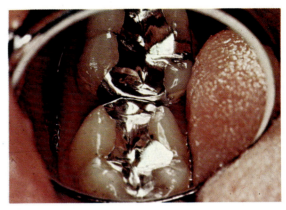

Polishing can be undertaken with a series of abrasive pastes of diminishing grit size, applied with a softened polishing brush (187); a final high lustre can be obtained with jeweller's rouge. Care must be taken not to overheat and create a false polish by drawing mercury to the surface. Alternatively a good polish can be created with

Baker-Curson finishing burs (see 177). Some people think that there is no benefit to be gained in polishing amalgam restorations but at least a polished filling will feel pleasantly smooth to the patient and its appearance will be satisfying to the operator (188).

189 After the initial carving of an amalgam restoration, close examination will often reveal 'feathers' of excess amalgam overlying the surface enamel (arrowed). This is most likely to happen when it has been decided not to eradicate all fissures or other surface irregularities. If left, these thin sections of amalgam will eventually fracture, leaving plaque retentive edges. Feathers of excess can be recognised readily if a mental image is retained of the original cavity outline (see 121).

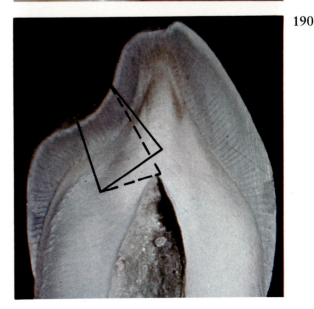

189

190 The imbalance between the size of cusps in a lower first premolar and the consequent position of the pulp requires a variation in the angulation of the occlusal lock and dovetail in these teeth (shown by the solid black line). Failure to appreciate this point can run the risk of a pulp exposure (indicated by the dotted line).

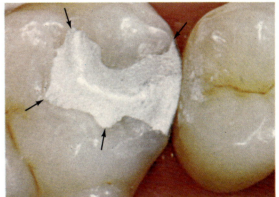

190

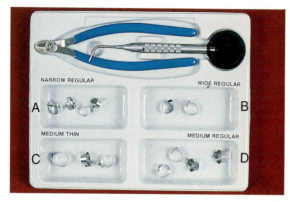

191

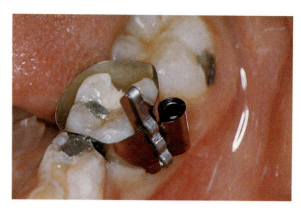

192

191, 192 When difficulty is experienced with a standard matrix band holder (for example the Bonnalie or Seqveland) a useful matrix to use is the Caulk's Automatrix (**191**), (L D Caulk Co., Milford, Delaware). This is a self-locking matrix which does away with the need for a matrix band holder (**192**); an advantage when retention of the matrix to the tooth is slight and the weight of the holder or mobility of the patient's lips keeps dislodging it.

The bands are supplied in a variety of widths and they are all capable of increasing their diameter to fit the largest of teeth (A, narrow regular; B, wide regular; C, medium thin; D, medium regular). A band is therefore chosen with a width sufficient to support the filling material from cervical floor to marginal ridge. It is readily slipped over the tooth and tightened by placing the end of the tightening tool into the roll of excess band material and rotating it until the band is firmly held.

To remove the band the top of the locking bracket is cut off with the blue handled cutters provided. These have a plastic cage attached to the cutting blades which catches the small metal fragment and prevents it from being swallowed or inhaled.

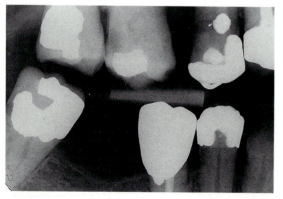

193

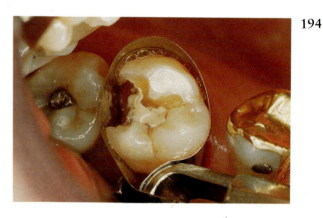

194

193–196 The area most vulnerable to recurrent caries in very extensive Class II restorations is at the cervical margin. It is often difficult to ensure the good adaptation of amalgam in such situations. Also the setting and temperature shrinkage of a large mass of amalgam are likely to break any cervical seal and consequently may aid the onset of recurrent caries. Removal of plaque in such inaccessible places is difficult even with dental floss.

For these reasons it is often advisable, where caries is well past the amelo-cemental junction (as seen distally in the upper second molar (**193**)) to use Ketac Silver for the deepest part of the box. First of all calcium hydroxide is placed over the pulpal aspects of the cavity for the usual reasons (**194**). Then Ketac Silver is packed well into the bottom 1–2 mm of the box (**195**) and allowed to set before topping off with amalgam (**196**) which provides a durable outer surface to the restoration.

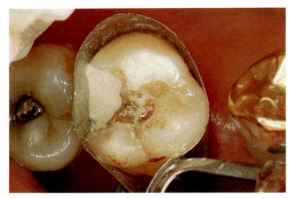

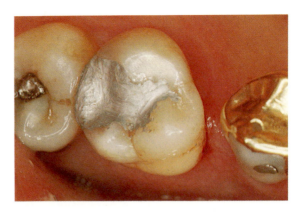

A similar approach, but for different reasons, is employed when a Class II posterior composite cavity is found to have a cervical margin placed on cementum rather than enamel. Composite adheres well to enamel using the the acid-etch technique whereas glass ionomer requires calcium to create a good seal (Shortall *et al.*, 1989), of which there is plenty in sound dentine and cementum.

Some faults in amalgam technique

197 A frequent observation, when examining amalgam restorations that have been in place for some time, is the 'ditching' effect around the margins. This is usually due to a fault at the butt-joint between amalgam and tooth. It can be due to the fracture and loss of enamel prisms, resulting from residual or recurrent caries. It is more likely, however, to be attributed to the fracture of an acute angle of amalgam at the restoration margin, created either by poor cavity design or over-contouring of the amalgam (Elderton, 1975). Creep and delayed amalgam expansion may also contribute towards weakening the amalgam margin. Mere marginal defects are not nowadays considered sufficient reason for total replacement of an amalgam restoration. If it is not associated with recurrent caries or discomfort from

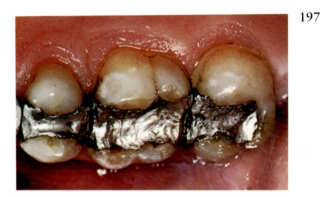

food trapping or a sharp margin it should not be touched but kept under observation. If recurrent caries has developed but on a small scale, a repair to the margin should be considered (see Chapter 20).

198 Recurrent caries can occur interproximally if the embrasure margins of a Class II restoration are not cleaned regularly. Cleansing used to be aided by extending the box walls to within the reach of the toothbrush bristles. In the modern, more conservative approach, the margins, if not accessible to the toothbrush, should be cleaned by meticulous flossing rather than by being extended unnecessarily. In this restoration the fault may have been in the poor finishing of the amalgam whose rough margins shredded the floss or prevented its application.

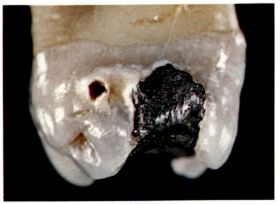

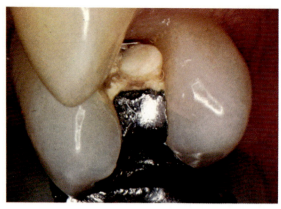

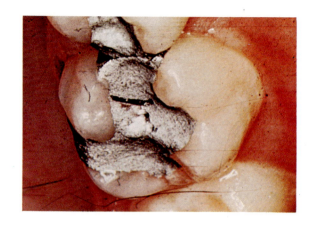

199 The loss of any restoration, in full or in part as shown here, should prompt a diagnosis as to the cause of the loss before a replacement is undertaken. Here the mesial box has broken from the rest of the amalgam restoration because of the lack of amalgam bulk in the keyway, or isthmus. This in turn was due to the use of too thick a base. Before replacing this filling, therefore, it is necessary to reduce the base to create space for an adequate bulk of amalgam. It might also be advisable to cut retention channels in the box cavity walls and to adjust the opposing cusp that might damage the new restoration.

200 A common finding where occlusal relationships were not checked carefully at the carving stage, is the burnished 'high spot'. The situation may be self adjusting by reduction through the wear of the excess amalgam. However, this process may cause unwelcome symptoms, such as tenderness of the tooth due to traumatic peridontitis or sensitivity due to pulpal hyperaemia. Furthermore, fracture of the filling may also occur as seen here. If occlusal relationships are such that the adjustments required would weaken the filling, then selective grinding of the opposing tooth could be justified. Such grinding should be followed by polishing the enamel with a paste containing fluoride.

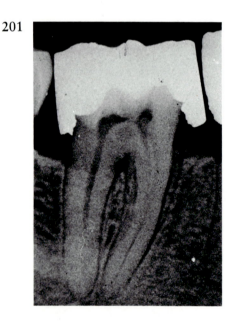

201 Failure to burnish the matrix band so that it mimics the external contours of the original tooth, together with a lack of cervical wedging, will result in a poorly contoured restoration with cervical excess as seen here. This will result in periodontal disease and possibly recurrent caries due to plaque retention and food packing. Another explanation of this poor contour could be that a copper ring had been used as the matrix.

202, 203 An unsightly amalgam tattoo (202) can be caused by the careless introduction of amalgam remnants into the socket of an extracted tooth if both an extraction and an amalgam restoration are undertaken at the same occasion. The amalgam could also simply have broken off an amalgam filling in the tooth being extracted. Only a small quantity of amalgam is required as the radiograph of the condition in the previous figure indicates (203).

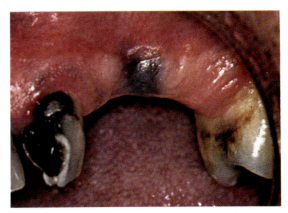

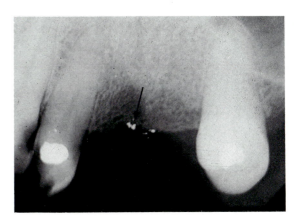

10 Composite and glass ionomer (polyalkenoate) cement restorations

Composite resins and glass ionomer (polyalkenoate) cements have superseded silicate cements. In the case of composites this is due to their superior physical properties, particularly strength and reduced solubility, and to their ability to bond to enamel. The problem of bonding composite to dentine has not yet been fully resolved. Much research in this field is under way, however, and several dentine bonding systems (see below) are available to the profession. It is perhaps too early to recommend them for routine use. Glass ionomers, on the other hand, through chemical bonding to calcium known as chelation, are able to adhere to both enamel and dentine and are relatively well tolerated by the pulp. Composites and glass ionomers are increasingly being used in new situations where this ability of retention to the enamel or dentine allows their application when no mechanical retention is available.

Dentine bonding agents

The structure of dentine compared with that of enamel does not lend itself readily to mechanical bonding of composites. There are also differences of chemical composition and the presence of tubules containing organic matter and moisture which further complicate the bonding mechanism.

Various methods have been adopted in order to overcome this problem. The smear layer of the dentine can be modified with an aqueous solution of HEMA and maleic acid prior to the placement of a bonding resin, containing mainly Bis-GMA and the final composite restoration (e.g. Scotchbond 2, 3M Company, Minnesota, USA).

Alternatively the bonding agent can adhere to the collagen of the dentine. In order for this to occur the smear layer is removed with EDTA before the dentine is coated with a primer and unfilled resin, after which the composite is placed (e.g. Gluma, Bayer Dental, Leverkusen, Germany).

However many of the systems available involve several stages of technique. One of the more simple is a light activated single component system which chemically alters the smear layer and chemically bonds to both enamel and dentine. The ready-mixed solution of methacrylate and carboxylic acid bonds to the calcium in the dentine whilst the methacrylate is available to bond to the composite restoration (e.g. Pertac Universal Bond, ESPE, Seefeld, Germany).

204 Before the advent of composites and glass ionomers, multiple Class V lesions were treated with unsightly amalgam or silicate, which soon became discoloured due to marginal staining.

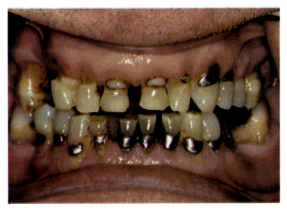

204

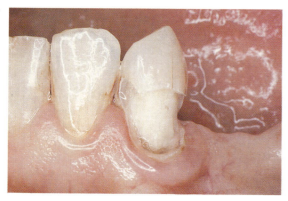

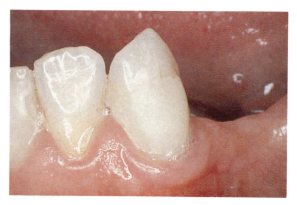

205, 206 Such Class V carious lesions and multiple cervical abrasion lesions can now be restored with glass ionomer cement, composite resin or a combination of both. In the abrasion defects shown in **24** there is an incomplete circumference of enamel and this precludes the use of composite on its own. Such lesions can readily be restored with glass ionomer (see **240**).

Glass ionomer however abrades easily, is soluble in oral fluids and is often poor aesthetically. These drawbacks can be overcome by using composite resin in conjunction with glass ionomer. When there is insufficient ·enamel or when good mechanical retention is difficult to obtain a substantial base of glass ionomer can be placed (**205**) which, together with any available enamel, gives satisfactory retention for the composite (**206**).

A composite tip restoration

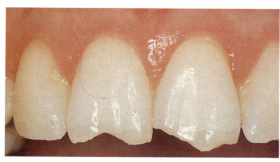

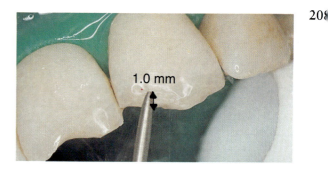

1.0 mm

207–221 The tips of these upper central incisors have been fractured (**207**). The teeth are not exposed and are vital. They are deemed suitable for restoration with acid-etched composite resin.

The periphery of the enamel is reduced to half thickness for a distance of one millimetre from the fractured margin (**208**). This can best be achieved with a high-speed bullet nose or torpedo diamond bur which will create a definitive chamfered finishing line to the preparation which is kept entirely in enamel (**209**, left and labial margin, right). A recognisable margin aids the accurate

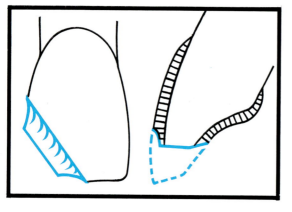

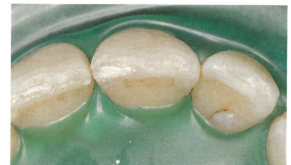

application of etchant gel and the trimming of composite excess. Furthermore, the shape of this reduction will allow a reasonable thickness of composite up to the restoration's margin. This is preferable to a feather edge finish, the bevel of which has the disadvantage that it may involve dentine (**209** right, palatal margin) thus reducing the amount of enamel available for retention.

The procedure is undertaken under rubber dam, whenever possible, to prevent contamination of the freshly cut and etched enamel with saliva which could seriously interfere with the union of composite to enamel.

The complete collar of reduced enamel can be seen in the incisal view of the incisors (**210**). Any exposed dentine is protected with a wash of acid resistant calcium hydroxide. A cellulose acetate crown form of appropriate shape is selected and trimmed so as just to overlap the surface enamel at the margin of the preparation (**211, 212**). When pressure is applied to the matrix margins, to adapt the composite, any excess can be reached and removed before being polymerised.

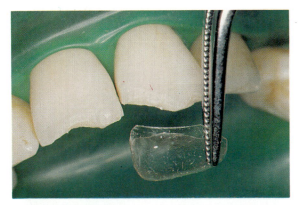

211

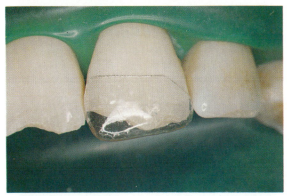

212

A pinhole is placed in the incisal/approximal corner of the matrix (**213**) to allow trapped air to escape when the composite is inserted, thus preventing the formation of a blow hole in the finished restoration.

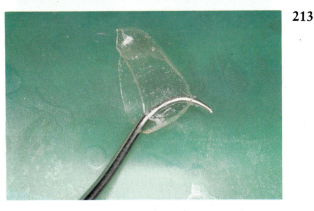

213

An etchant in coloured gel form is applied for 30–60 seconds to the prepared enamel (**214**) with a small brush or sponge pledget. The etchant should then be thoroughly washed off with a vigorous water spray and the etched surface dried and examined for successful etching. This is recognised by the chalky appearance of etched enamel (**215**) caused by the differential removal of enamel crystals and the formation of micropores (see **57**).

214

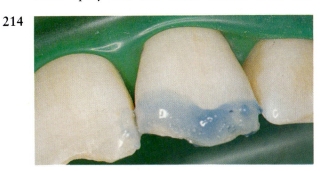

215

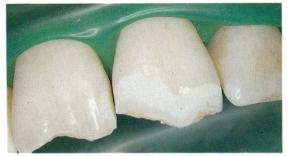

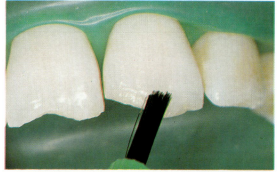
216

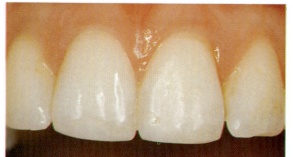
217

Unfilled resin is painted onto the etched enamel (216) and the excess dissipated with a gentle air stream before polymerising with 15 seconds application of light. Care should be taken not to blow excess resin into inaccessible places, such as interproximally or subgingivally, where it would be difficult to remove after polymerisation.

If rubber dam is used the shade of the tooth should have been taken prior to its application as the tooth will lighten as it dries out. The correct shade of composite is loaded into the crown form. A small extrusion of composite from the pinhole is evidence of the complete evacuation of any trapped air (217).

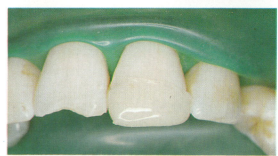
218

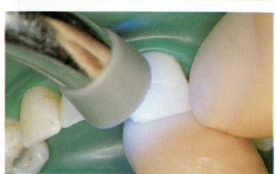
219

The loaded matrix is applied to the tooth ensuring correct placement for a good contact point and cervical adaptation (218). To achieve the latter it may be advisable to insert a wooden wedge. Polymerisation is then activated with a curing light for 40 seconds (219). To ensure that all portions are fully cured it is advisable to apply the light for a further period to all areas that may have been masked by the fingers.

Any shaping or removal of positive edges of composite can be accomplished with a flexible disc manufactured for this purpose (220). The best surface finish is that left by the matrix but, if the restoration has to be reduced, the high gloss can be restored with the finest of the flexible discs or special rubber cups and points. Where access for any of these is impossible, Baker-Curson burs can be used. The resulting restorations are best assessed by patient and operator when the rubber dam is removed (221). This will also allow the occlusion to be checked both in intercuspal and protrusive positions.

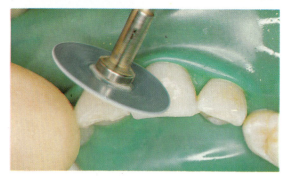
220

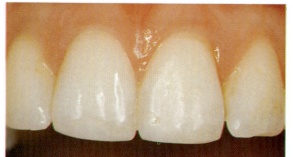
221

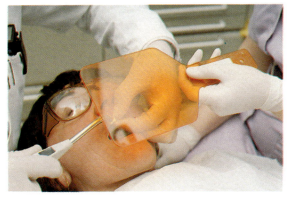

222 The intense light emitted by the curing lamp can be harmful to the eyes of both the operator and chairside assistant. Use of a hand held filter will protect the eyes whilst still allowing the dentist to see the operating area.

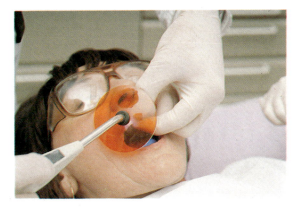

223 For single handed working the filter can be attached to the working end of the curing lamp.

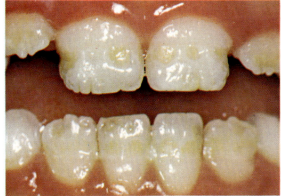

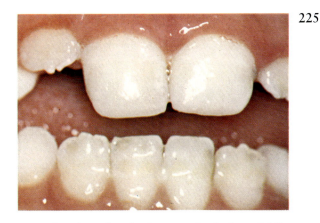

224, 225 This is an example of enamel hypoplasia (**224**) where the upper central incisors have been treated with acid-etched composite facings (**225**).

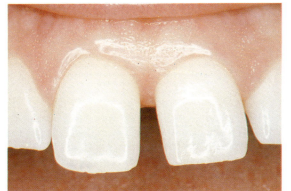

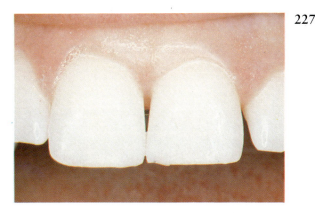

226, 227 Composite can be applied to the tips and interproximal surfaces of perfectly sound teeth if some change in their shape is required, for instance, to close the diastema as seen here.

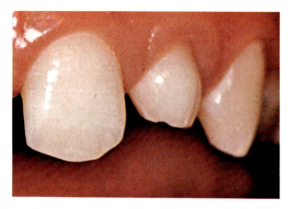

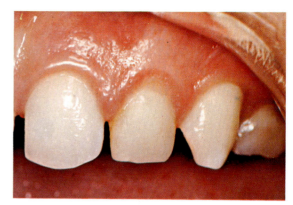

228, 229 This young patient has hypodontia with missing lateral incisors and a retained primary canine (**228**). The appearance of the retained primary tooth has been made to resemble a permanent lateral incisor by use of an acid-etched composite facing (**229**), shown here 12 months after insertion.

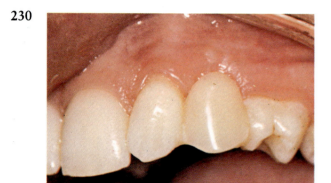

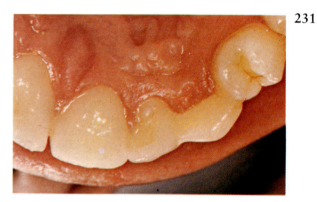

230, 231 The acid-etch technique can be used in an emergency to attach a temporary pontic to an adjacent tooth. Here a stock acrylic denture tooth has been trimmed to fit the upper canine space. It is attached with composite to the acid-etched surfaces of the neighbouring teeth. Provided the pontic is not subjected to heavy occlusal loading it will constitute a very convenient stop gap for a patient who has lost a denture or who is awaiting the construction of a bridge.

Composite restorations in posterior teeth

The case for the use of composite in place of amalgam for Class II restorations has not yet been convincingly made. Most operators will accept that composite has a role in restoring small lesions, particularly those which would involve loss of sound tooth tissue to provide retention for amalgam. Many operators, however still have reservations about using composite in larger lesions, particularly those with adequate retention for amalgam, or in sites of particular occlusal stress, because the resulting wear of the composite may allow over-eruption or forward drift of the restored tooth. On the other hand the occasional use of composite in the very large Class II cavity can be recommended because its adhesive properties are capable of holding weakened cusps in place which might otherwise fracture if amalgam were to be used. If a tooth is already exhibiting signs of 'cracked tooth syndrome' then a composite may be the best choice short of molar endodontics, a full coverage crown or indeed extraction.

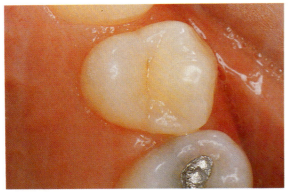

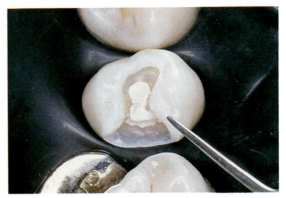

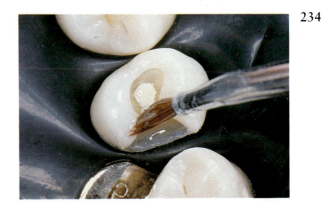

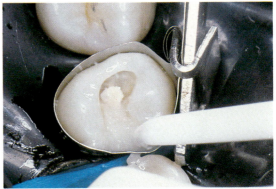

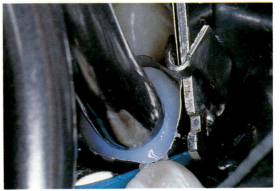

232–239 There are always the wishes or even demands of the patients for 'white fillings' to be considered, particularly in the more obvious premolar teeth (**232**) when aesthetic considerations may overrule all others.

After removal of the amalgam from this premolar the cavity floor is lined with calcium hydroxide and the enamel walls etched (**233**). It should be noted that although in an anterior composite restoration the occlusal enamel would be bevelled no attempt has been made to do so here. This is because wear or fracture of a thin margin could lead to a deficient restoration.

Following etching, unfilled resin is painted on the enamel (**234**) and polymerised with 15 seconds application of the curing light.

Initially only the cervical half of the cavity box is packed with composite (**235**) care being taken to ensure full adaptation to the cervical floor and box corners before polymerisation (**236**). A layered technique of filling is required for two basic reasons. Firstly the curing light is only effective through 2-3 mm of composite. To pack to a greater depth risks leaving the gingival portion unpolymerised. Secondly, if too great a mass is polymerised at a time, the resulting polymerisation shrinkage is likely to pull the composite from its attachment to the cervical layer of resin. It is a sensible precaution to apply more light to the cervical margin from both buccal and palatal sides after the matrix band has been removed. Alternatively a transparent matrix can be used with perspex wedges to which the light can be applied first to make sure that polymerisation is initiated at and towards the vulnerable cervical margin.

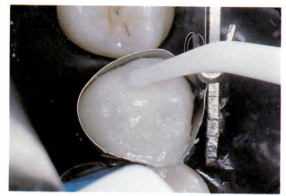

237

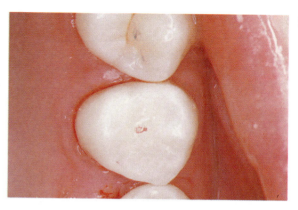

23

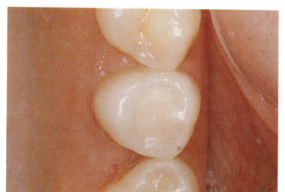

239

Filling of the cavity is completed, shaping the composite as closely as possible to the required occlusal contours (**237**) before final polymerisation. This will save considerable time at the finishing stage. After removal of the dam it is essential to check carefully for the absence of occlusal interference using the finest of articulating paper e.g. GHM. Composite is a most unyielding material and if a high spot exists it will not be self-adjusting as can be the case with amalgam and could give rise to considerable discomfort. Here a small interference is revealed (**238**) in the centre of the occlusal surface.

Final adjustments can be made to any positive margins at a subsequent visit (**239**) provided they do not constitute interferences or roughness. Note how the colour of the teeth has recovered from the desiccation suffered under the rubber dam.

A glass ionomer (polyalkenoate) restoration

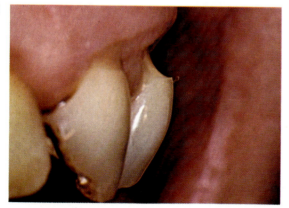

240

240–243 The cementum and dentine in the labial cervical region of this tooth have been seriously abraded by the toothbrush (**240**). It is difficult, and unwarranted, to create a retentive cavity in such a situation.

There is insufficient enamel to retain a composite restoration and this form of lesion presents the ideal situation for a glass ionomer restoration because of its ability to adhere to dentine.

No cavity preparation of the dentine is required if it is not carious but it must be cleaned and conditioned to present calcium ions at the surface to allow chelation with the glass ionomer. This can be done with dilute citric acid or polyacrylic acid.

The glass ionomer is mixed to a stiff consistency and its application to the tooth can be aided by a cervical foil, the margins of which are closely burnished to the surrounding tooth. Such a foil will provide a good contour (**241**).

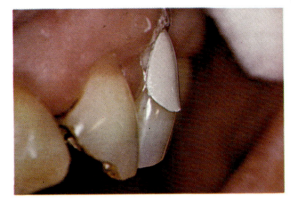

241

The excess cement can be removed before it sets so that on removal of the foil very little trimming should be required. The surface of the ionomer should be protected with a varnish or a film of polymerised composite resin before there is any chance of moisture contamination. Any trimming is best postponed until a subsequent visit. This can best be undertaken with a Baker-Curson bur whilst the gingival margin is retracted to a safe position with a flat plastic instrument (**242**).

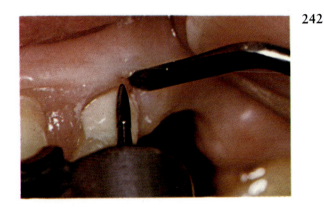

242

The resulting restoration in this case (**243**) has quite an acceptable colour match. If however the shade presents a problem, a covering of matching composite can be used in a 'sandwich' technique.

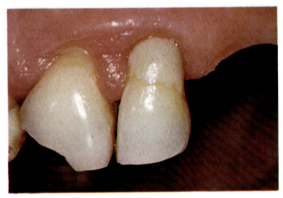

243

11 Aids to retention

When caries has destroyed or undermined tooth tissue extensively there is the problem of gaining retention for a restoration from the sound tissue that remains. Where possible, the standard retentive devices such as dovetails and undercuts should first be incorporated into the cavity form. These may, however, be insufficient in which case retention may be supplemented by the use of pins, posts or retentive channels. Pins are inserted into the vital dentine around which the plastic filling material, usually amalgam or composite, is packed. In non-vital root-filled teeth advantage may be taken of the existence of natural holes, the pulp canals, as posts can be fitted to these. A more recent development is to place undercut slots in the dentine of the cavity floor into which amalgam is packed (Newsome, 1988). These restorations may be successful without the provision of a full veneer crown but they should be periodically monitored for premature failure.

The approach to the problems of retention can be demonstrated by consideration of a series of cavity preparations for lesions of increasing sizes.

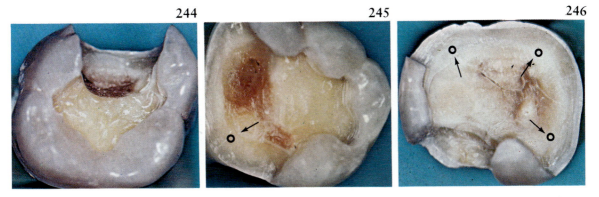

244   245   246

244 In this molar there was a large interproximal carious lesion dealt with by a cavity preparation which has produced a large, wide box. Occlusal extension into buccal and lingual fissures has, however, provided a satisfactory retentive dovetail and further retention from pins should not be required.

246 This very extensive preparation leaves little sound tissue to support the restoration. Some retention form has been created with a buccal box which was necessary to deal with the caries involving the buccal fissure. Applying the 'rule of thumb' that one pin should be used for every cusp that is missing, three pins will be needed here as indicated. This rule will need to be adjusted, up or down, according to the likely stress that will be applied to the restoration.

245 The caries in this lower first molar has been more extensive than that in the previous example and this has caused loss of the mesio-lingual cusp. Some retention form has been achieved from a dovetail cut into the distal end of the occlusal surface but this is probably insufficient for successful retention. It should therefore be supplemented with a pin in the position marked with an arrow.

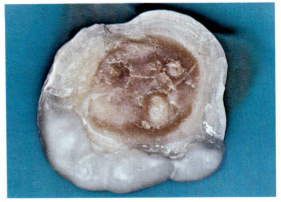

247

247 No retention form was feasible in this example. The sound buccal wall provides some resistance form and a buccal box is not justified here. Four pins will be needed.

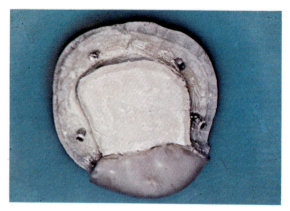

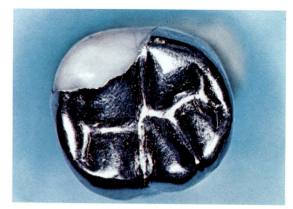

248 This example, similar in extent to the previous figure, shows four pins in position. A base has been inserted to reduce the size of the amalgam to reasonable proportions. Care has been taken to keep the base clear of the pins so that the amalgam may be condensed all round them for maximum grip.

249 An amalgam restoration may be retained exclusively by pins and carved to restore fully the original crown anatomy. In many mouths a restoration such as this may well stand up to normal wear and tear. However should it not the amalgam may be reduced at a later date to act as a core for the support of a full veneer gold crown (see **316, 317**).

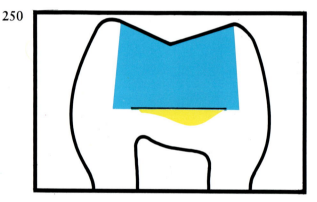

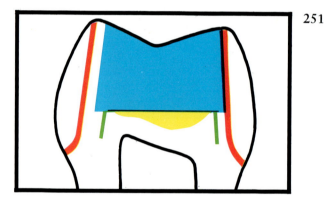

250, 251 Pin retention may be advisable for any tooth requiring a large amalgam if there is the possibility of a subsequent crown being required. This is still the case even if pinning is not considered essential for the retention of the initial amalgam (**250**). This is to anticipate the weakening of the remaining tooth tissue (**251**) following full crown preparation. This reduction might remove much, or all, of the support for the amalgam core which would then need to rely almost totally on pins for its retention.

Types of pin for supplementary retention

The simplest form of extra retention is obtained by drilling a hole in the dentine with a narrow flat fissure bur and cementing into this a short length of stainless steel orthodontic wire. Retention of the amalgam to such pins can be increased by bending the protruding portion. A refinement of the cemented pin is to use threaded wire which gives better grip both to the cement and the amalgam.

Cemented pins are of value when no other sort is available but they have been superseded by more precise systems of self-tapping pins, a considerable range of which has been developed by the manufacturers.

252 Self-tapping pins screw into slightly undersize pinholes that are cut into the dentine with a twist drill. Provided they are inserted in a forward rotatory direction they will cut their own thread into dentine and thus give considerably more retention than cement.

One such system is the Thread-Mate-System (TMS, Whaledent International, NY - NY, USA) which has a choice of pin and twist drill sizes ranging up, as shown here from left to right, from Minikin, Minim to Regular. Some of the pins are supplied as '2 in 1' with a shearing point half way along the double length pin. The twist drills are shouldered for safety thus preventing the pinhole from being made dangerously deep. The length of most pins available is 4mm with a twist drill length of 2mm. Thus the pin, if properly inserted, will provide 2mm of grip in the dentine and 2mm in the amalgam.

253 TMS pins are inserted in a variety of ways, either manually by a finger held driver (left) or by use of a handpiece held chuck (middle) or bur adaptor (right). A system which allows insertion of a pin by handpiece has a distinct advantage in that if access has been possible to drill the pinhole it is equally possible to insert the pin. This is not always the case when hand chucks or spanners are used. The TMS pin is bendable after insertion and it is gold plated to resist corrosion.

254 Other systems such as Stabilok (Fairfax Dental Ltd., London, UK) as shown, and Filpin (S.J. Filhol Dental Mfg. Co. Ltd. West Cork, Ireland) provide the pin and bur shank in one piece. The shouldered twist drill will cut a pinhole in the dentine to a depth equal to half the pin length. The pin is driven into the pinhole until it shears off the shank on meeting the bottom of the hole. The pins are bendable and the Stabilok pins are supplied in two sizes of diameter.

Pin retention – posterior teeth

255–267 The cutting of pinholes into dentine is not without risk and should not be undertaken lightly. The main risk is that the pinhole may be drilled off course and penetrate into the periodontal ligament or the pulp chamber (**255**).

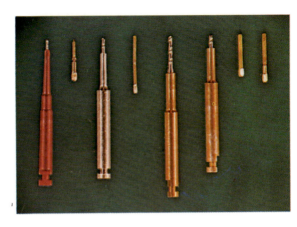

252

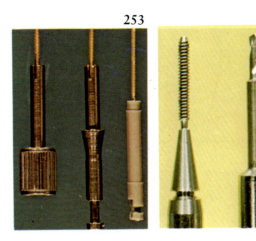

253 254

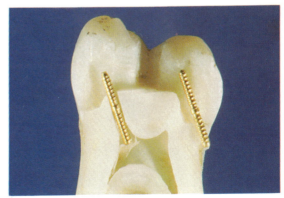

255

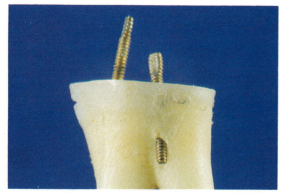

256

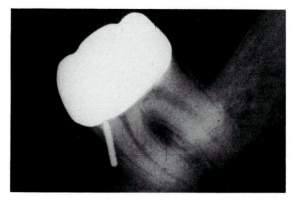

257

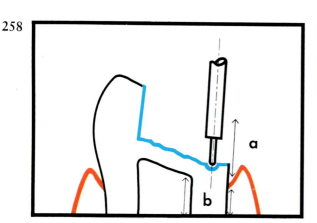

258

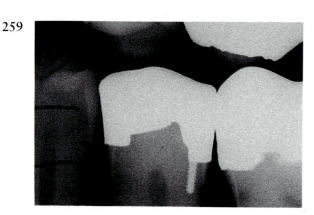

259

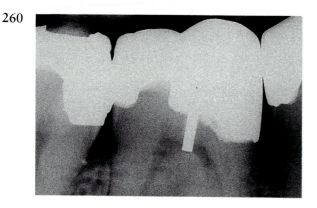

260

The periodontal ligament is particularly vulnerable if the pinhole is drilled immediately over a bifurcation or trifurcation (256) or if due allowance is not made for a tilted tooth (257). A further risk is that the enamel may fracture from the side of the pinhole if it is placed along the amelo-dentinal junction. It is therefore important to assess carefully the anatomical situation before preparing any pinholes, firstly to decide the starting point and secondly to decide the direction in which it should be cut. It is helpful to create a depression in the dentine with a small round bur as a starting pit for each hole. Such a pit will keep the twist hole to its intended access point. This should be 1mm inside the amelo-dentinal or cemento-dentinal junction (see 297) and away from the furcation zones

The direction of the pinhole should be parallel to the inner and outer surfaces of the dentine into which it is placed (258). This direction can be assessed by placing a probe against the accessible root surface (a) and, for mesial and distal pinholes, by studying a bitewing radiograph (b).

Bitewing radiographs should always be consulted when placing pins mesially or distally to ensure correct angulation of the pin (259). Pins placed buccally or lingually however will be superimposed on the pulp chamber and their angulation in a pulpal/periodontal direction cannot be seen radiographically (260).

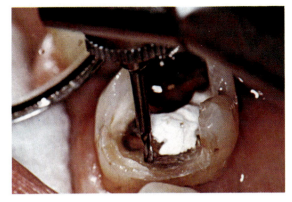

261

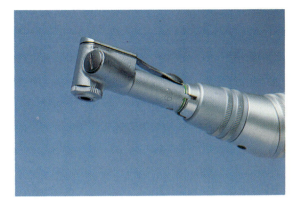

262

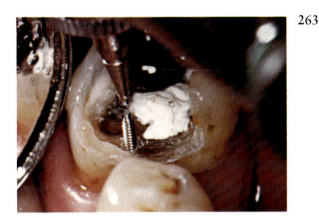

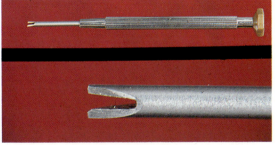

263

264

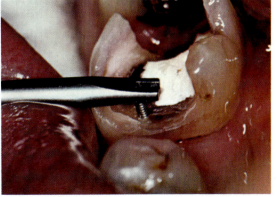

265

To cut the pinhole the twist drill is placed in the starting pit and carefully lined up in the predetermined direction (261). The hole is cut to the depth of the drill's shoulder, preferably in one go. This is to avoid deviation from the intended direction that might otherwise occur. If more than one attempt is required to complete the cutting great care should be exercised to maintain the original direction of cut. It should be appreciated that there is a risk of over-enlarging the pinhole each time the drill is re-inserted. For this reason it is advisable to use the smaller diameter twist drill and pin of the two sizes supplied by Stabilok. If this pinhole inadvertently gets over size or is spoilt by inserting the pin in the reverse direction of rotation, the operator can fall back on the larger size and start again. If the pin will still not self-tap it may have to be cemented if there is no alternative site in which it can be placed.

On no account must the drill be allowed to stall in the hole. It will be impossible to restart the motor and attempts to remove the drill will almost inevitably cause it to break.

To insert the self-shearing pin it is recommended that a speed reduction head (262) be used to increase the torque of the modern dental motor and to reduce the risk of damage to the thread cut in the dentine by insertion at too great a speed. The speed reduction head should be allowed to reach maximum motor revs before the pin is pushed into the pinhole. The actual pin speed will of course be much less. The pin will tap itself into the dentine and come to a sudden stop at the bottom of the pinhole when the momentum of the dental motor will cause the pin to shear from its shank (263).

If it proves necessary, the pin may be bent. This can be done most safely with a special tool (264) which can turn the outer end of the pin (265) without putting heavy stress on the retaining dentine.

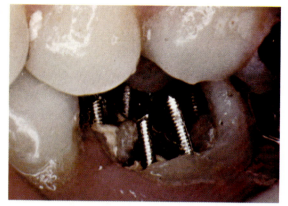

266

The length and direction of the external part of each pin should be checked for adequate clearance between the pin and the opposing teeth (**266**). If the pins are not visible when the teeth are in occlusion the required clearance of 1mm can be checked by getting the patient to bite on a softened piece of 1mm thick prosthetic wax. If the pin leaves no imprint on the wax, clearance is sufficient.

If it may become necessary to cover the pinned amalgam with a gold crown it is advisable to bend the pins well inwards (**267**) to avoid them being laid bare or even cut off during the preparation for the full veneer crown.

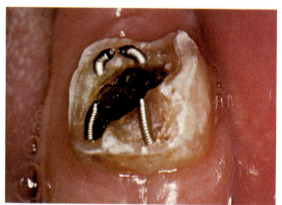

267

268 A useful alternative to self-tapping pins is the use of undercut slots placed in the floor of a large amalgam cavity. If the tooth to be filled is also root-filled, advantage can be taken of this by packing amalgam into the chamber previously occupied by the pulp. This is particularly applicable to the large pulp chambers of molar teeth. In this example the traditional principles of cavity preparation have been applied.

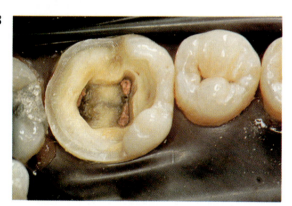

268

269 Slots are introduced into the cervical floor of the cavity with a slow speed small inverted cone bur which will ensure that the slots have retentive undercuts. The slots themselves should be positioned equidistant between the pulp chamber and the root surface.

270 The final restoration may well survive perfectly well as an amalgam restoration but if required it will also provide a very retentive core for a full veneer crown.

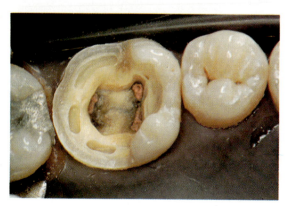

269

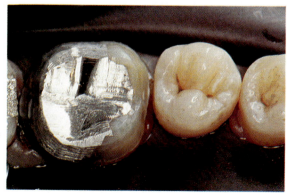

270

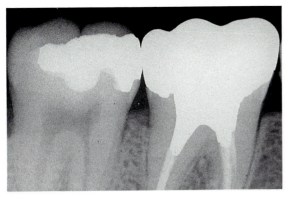

271

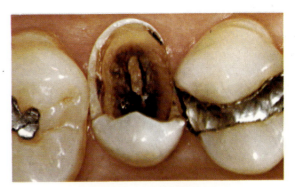

272

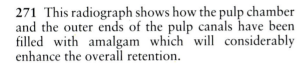

273

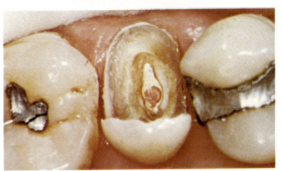

274

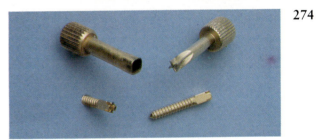

275

271 This radiograph shows how the pulp chamber and the outer ends of the pulp canals have been filled with amalgam which will considerably enhance the overall retention.

272–275 If the tooth to be restored is a root-filled premolar, which is not usually suited to the slot technique just described, it may be preferable to gain retention via a post in the root canal rather than further weaken the remaining tooth tissue with a series of pinholes. This example is of a single rooted upper second premolar, root-filled and with extensive caries which has left only the palatal cusp standing (**272**). After caries and unsupported enamel have been removed the gutta percha root filling can be seen (**273**).

Retention can be obtained by removal of the coronal half of the root filling and by shaping the canal to receive a parallel-sided threaded screw post such as the Svedia or Nordin post (Svedia International, CH-1817 Brent, Montreux) seen here (**274**) with driver and box spanner which are used for insertion. The canal is shaped with an engine reamer to an accurate size for self-tapping the post into place. There is a range of posts of different diameters with reamers (**275**) to match the six post sizes.

276 The procedure, shown on another tooth, is to remove gutta percha and root filling sealer with a round steel or a Gates Glidden bur and make room for the access of the Svedia engine reamer.

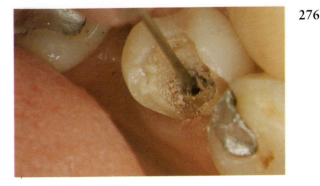

276

277

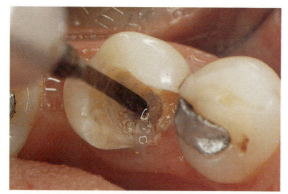

278

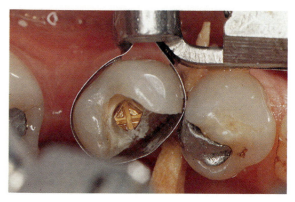

279

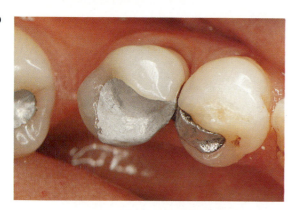

280

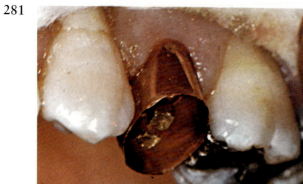

281

277 The size of engine reamer chosen should be just larger in diameter than the post hole created by the Gates Glidden bur. The post hole is then reamed to an appropriate length, that is to say long enough to give secure retention but not too long to jeopardise the remaining root filling.

278 The Svedia post is then inserted with a driver which self-taps it into the slightly undersize post hole. Care must be taken not to screw the post too far as this would risk splitting the root (see 290). It is then unscrewed to allow insertion of cement before finally screwing home. The combination of tapping into sound dentine and cementing gives retention of a very high order to posts of this type.

279 The application of a well wedged matrix ensures a well condensed amalgam. Care should be taken with the carving to reduce the occlusal surface in areas of possible heavy contact with opposing teeth.

280–283 In a two-rooted premolar it is possible to increase retention by the insertion of two posts, one in each canal (280).

 Where little or no crown tissue remains a copper band may be preferred for a matrix (281). If amalgam is to be the core material the band may be left in place until the patient's next visit. This will prevent damage to the amalgam by early removal of the matrix or by mastication before the amalgam has fully set.

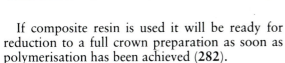

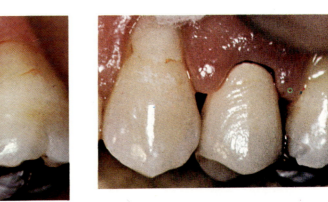

If composite resin is used it will be ready for reduction to a full crown preparation as soon as polymerisation has been achieved (282).

This twin post technique overcomes the problem associated with the provision of a post crown for a two rooted premolar and has provided the core for a bonded porcelain crown (283). The gingival condition would be expected to improve rapidly now that the potential for plaque retention has been considerably reduced by a good fitting crown and the use of porcelain.

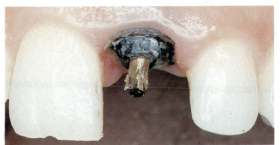

284 It is possible to use a threaded post, as seen here, in the provision of an anterior post crown. This is particularly useful when the root of the tooth being crowned is not long enough to give sufficient retention for a cast and cemented post, (see post crowns).

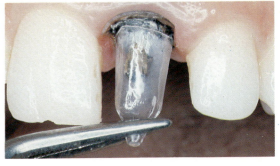

285 A Kerr's Coreform (Kerr Manufacturing Co., Emeryville, Ca., USA.) can be selected and trimmed to fit over the protruding part of the screw post.

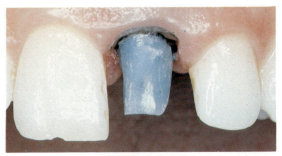

286 After filling with composite the crown form is re-inserted. When polymerised this composite core, probably with little further adjustment, will create a jacket crown preparation ready for impressions.

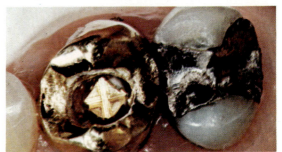

287 It is sometimes found that a tooth has lost its vitality after it has been restored by a full veneer crown. Root canal therapy then has to be performed through an access hole in the occlusal surface of the crown. After completion of the root filling it may be advisable to ensure the future retention of the crown by using supplementary retention, as it were in retrospect, by fitting a screw post to the root canal.

288

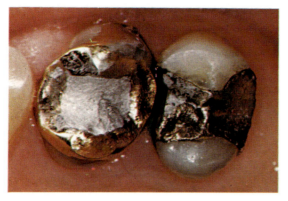

288 The access hole can then be packed with amalgam to complete the retention between the crown and post.

289

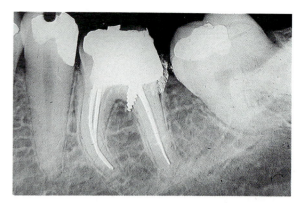

289 Screw posts are not without their dangers.and careful prior assessment followed by meticulous technique are essential if problems are to be avoided. In this example the reamed hole did not follow the original pulp canal, the reamer possibly being deflected by the silver point used for root filling. The resulting perforation into the bifurcation area has seriously compromised the prognosis for this tooth.

290

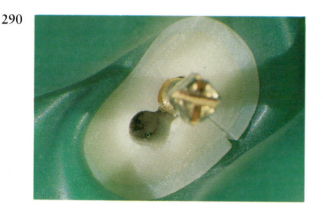

290, 291 Longitudinal root fractures are a real risk if tapered posts are used or if a post is screwed into place too tightly.

291

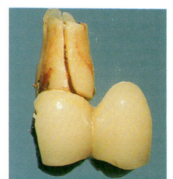

292

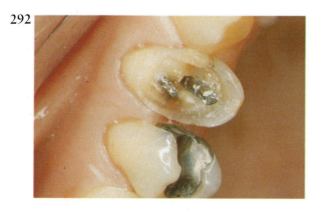

292, 293 If the risk of root splitting by self-tapping is considered to be too great, a close fitting cemented post may be used instead. The stainless steel Parapost (Whaledent International, NY - NY, USA.) seen here is cemented into a post hole cut with a matching Parapost reamer. It is often wise to

293

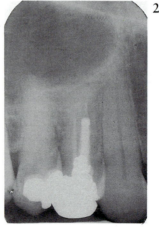

add a dentine screw pin in such situations to reduce the risk of dislodgement by torque stresses that may be applied to the finished crown.

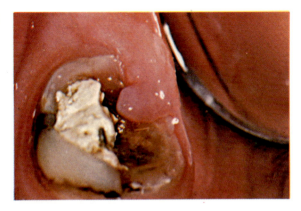

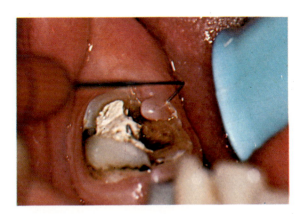

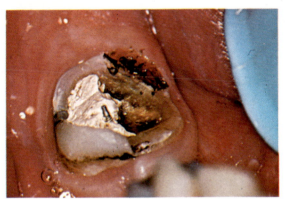

294–296 Gum tissue may be found to have proliferated over the cervical margin of a broken down tooth (**294**) and before a pinned amalgam can conveniently be placed this excess tissue needs to be removed. This can most easily be accomplished with the surgical diathermy which makes a clean incision (**295**) and leaves a dry field. The high speed suction nozzle performs the dual task of tissue retraction and evacuation of the smell of burning tissue before it is detected by the patient. Care must be taken not to let the sucker create too dry a field or this will interfere with the effectiveness of the diathermy.

The resultant wound being a dry one (**296**) allows work to continue on the restoration of this tooth without delay.

Pin retention – anterior teeth

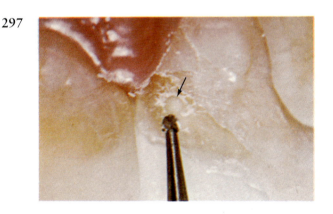

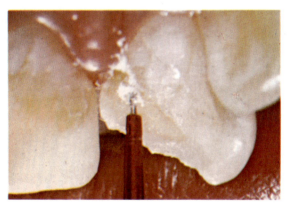

297–301 The retention provided for large anterior composites by acid-etching to enamel is usually more than adequate. However in excessively large restorations where there may be insufficient enamel it may be decided to supplement the retention of an anterior composite tip restoration with a pin. The Minikin pin, the smallest in the TMS range is specially designed for this purpose. The starting pit is placed with a small round bur (**297**) and the pinhole is drilled with the twist drill (**298**) that

299

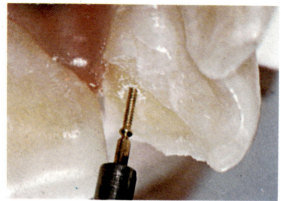

300

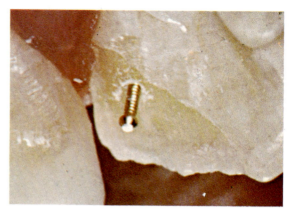

301

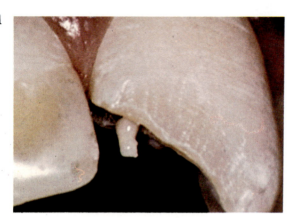

matches the Minikin pin. The easy access to anterior teeth allows the use of a finger driver to insert the pin (**299**).

The Minikin has a small mushroom shaped head for extra retention (**300**) and its gold plating is a precaution against discolouration from corrosion which could show through the semi-translucency of the completed filling. The pin itself may however show through and to disguise this its labial side should be painted with opaque composite (**301**) before the application of the main bulk of composite.

302

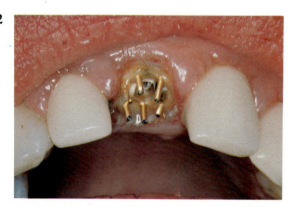

302, 303 Pins may also provide the only means of placing a crown in a case when the original post crown has fractured leaving the post in the root. If the broken post cannot be removed to allow a remake of the post crown the only solution is to obtain retention with several dentine pins (**302**) placed so as to give retention for composite that can be trimmed into a jacket crown preparation (**303**).

303

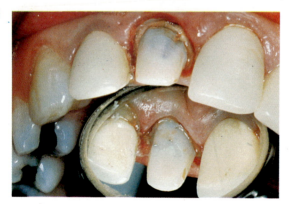

12 Posterior indirect restorations

Intra-coronal restorations

Restorations which are placed into non-undercut cavities cut into enamel and dentine, and which receive support and retention from the surrounding tooth tissue, are classed as inlays or intra-coronal restorations. Many of the principles that cover the traditional amalgam cavity preparations apply also to inlay cavity preparation, including outline form, resistance form and removal of carious dentine. Any differences are related to the fact that the inlay is constructed out of the mouth and thus has to be capable of insertion into the cavity, and that, if the inlay is to be constructed in gold, the margins have to be capable of being burnished to cover over the cement lute. These differences resolve themselves into two aspects of cavity preparation – the cavity walls and the cavity margins.

In order that a wax pattern may be removed from the tooth or its replica - the die - the walls of the cavity must be free from undercuts. The same freedom from undercuts permits the insertion of the cast inlay into the tooth. Linked with this consideration, however, is the need to supply retention for the restoration which in the amalgam cavity was provided by undercuts. This is gained by so angling the walls of the cavity that they are as near parallel to the line of insertion of the inlay as convenience will allow - usually quoted as 5° to the line of withdrawal or, put another way, 10° between opposing cavity walls. Retention is then described as being a function of the length and the near-parallelism of these walls.

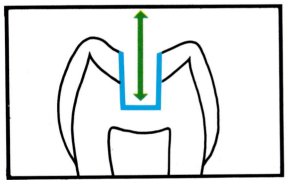

304

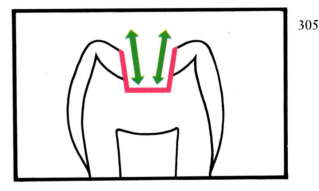

305

304, 305 In these illustrations the retention for the cavity drawn in blue is good, having near parallel walls and a long, single line of insertion (in green). The retention of the cavity, drawn in magenta, is poor due to walls that diverge more than is desirable and a shallow floor, both factors contributing to short and multiple lines of insertion (in green).

306–309 Good though the retention of an inlay may be, it still requires to be cemented in place. This is to resist removal of the inlay in a direction opposite to that of its insertion, for instance by a sticky toffee. Between the inlay and the cavity therefore is interposed a film of cement which, being soluble in mouth fluids, will eventually wash out and leave a gap between inlay and enamel margin. To prevent, or greatly reduce, any serious consequences arising from this situation, advantage is taken of the strength and malleability

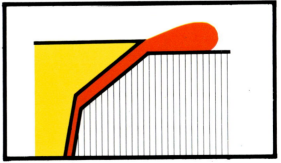

306

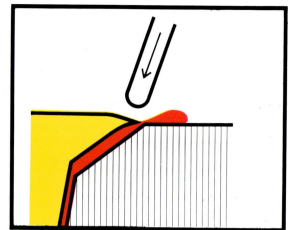

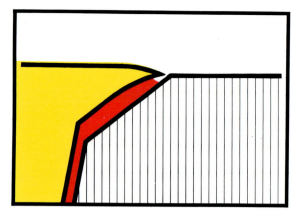

of gold which will allow a thin margin to be bent (burnished) into contact with the enamel and thus cover over the cement lute.

To be thin enough to allow burnishing, the angle of the gold margin must be 45° or less. This implies a cavo-surface angle of 135° or more.

Immediately after insertion a sectional view of the inlay and the cavity margin would show a marginal gap equivalent to the film thickness of the cement (306).

Preliminary burnishing before the cement has set will reduce the marginal film thickness of the cement to a minimum (307). At a later visit, when the superficial layer of cement has been leached out by the oral fluids (308), the burnishing can be completed to bring the gold margin into contact with the enamel (309). If this is done with a finishing bur or stone it is important that the direction of rotation of the bur (thin arrows) should be from gold towards enamel and that the handpiece itself is also moved only in this same direction (thick arrows). Some slight thinning of the gold, as indicated in green, will assist the burnishing process and the result should be a flush margin to the inlay that is barely detectable to a probe.

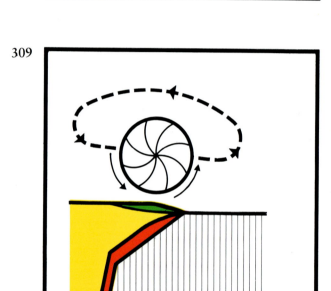

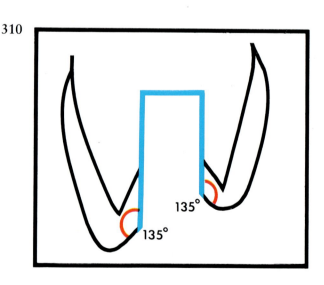

310 Where the cusps are steep the required 135° cavo-surface line angle may already exist as shown here. With flatter cusps, in molars and attrited teeth for instance, and at cervical margins, a bevel needs to be added to create the desired angle. This can be done smoothly and delicately with Baker-Curson tungsten carbide burs of appropriate shape (see 177).

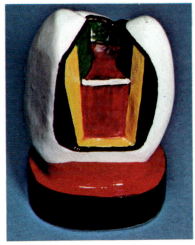

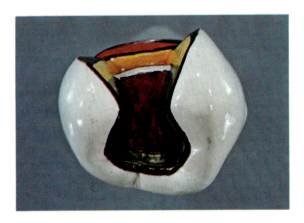

312 An occlusal view of the previous figure emphasises the withdrawal/insertion form. All the surfaces of the cavity walls can be seen from a single viewing point above the cavity. This can be an effective clinical test for absence of undercuts provided that one eye is closed to allow only monocular vision. The fact that the walls are only just visible is confirmation that near-parallelism has been obtained. The final test for freedom from undercuts can be made with a straight probe held in the direction of withdrawal and moved to touch each cavity wall in turn or by a trial wax pattern.

311 This interproximal view of a single box Class II gold inlay cavity shows in green the retentive form achieved occlusally and, in yellow, the retentive form of the box. The bevelling is depicted in dark blue; that of the box walls being most precisely applied with a disc if access allows. The white line shows the internal bevelling of the pulpo-axial line angle.

Extra-coronal restorations

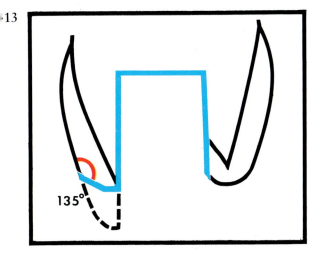

313 Occlusal coverage may be required for an inlay cavity where one or more of the cusps is weak. This 'capping' of the cusp is achieved by the reduction of the cusp height to give approximately 1.0mm clearance from the opposing tooth followed by the addition of a 'reverse' bevel to achieve the usual cavo-surface line angle of 135°. The inlay will thus cover the cusp and protect it from occlusal stress.

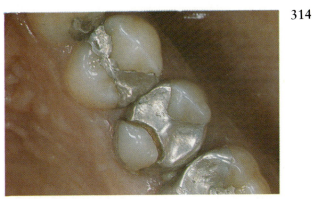

314 The palatal cusp of this upper second premolar, weakened by the occlusal width of the cavity, might not have fractured if a gold restoration with cuspal protection had been used instead of amalgam.

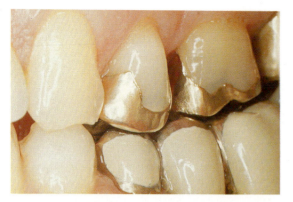

315 By virtue of its strength, gold can be used entirely extra-coronally and thus completely protect what remains of the crown of the tooth. Such crowns may be $^5/_8$, $^3/_4$ or full coverage or full veneer crowns and can be made in yellow gold or, should aesthetics demand it, platinised gold which can be faced with porcelain bonded directly to the metal.

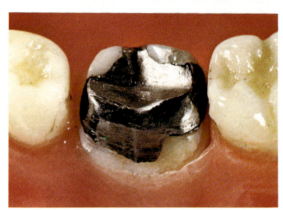

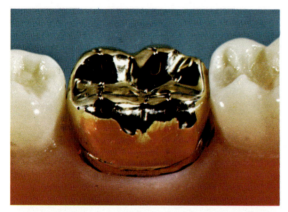

316, 317 Teeth requiring full veneer crowns usually do so because of extensive caries, although an abutment tooth required as a support for a bridge might be only minimally carious or even caries-free. When grossly carious, the first step in providing a full crown must be to remove all carious dentine and weakened enamel. This tissue must then be replaced with a plastic filling material, preferably amalgam, suitably retained by pins, posts or grooves (see Chapter 11).

The rebuilt crown is then prepared to allow room for coverage with metal, taking note of the need for near-parallelism, freedom from undercuts, occlusal clearance and correct marginal finish (**316**). The full veneer crown can then replicate the external dimensions and shape of the original tooth as seen here (**317**).

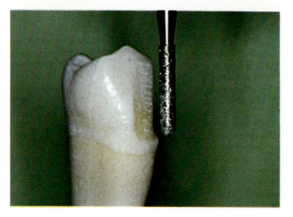

318–324 The appropriate marginal finish for a full veneer crown preparation is what might be termed a 135° chamfer. The advantages of this are that only a minimal amount of tooth tissue is removed compared with a shouldered preparation and yet, a more easily recognisable margin can be seen on a die compared with a feather edge.

This 135° chamfer is readily prepared using a bullet or torpedo shaped diamond bur (**318**) or tungsten bur. The shape and dimensions of such a bur ensure that adequate reduction and near-parallelism are achieved at the same time as the correct margin is being created, provided that

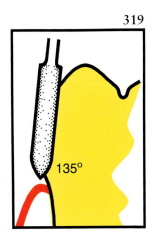

319

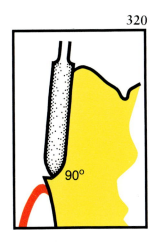

320

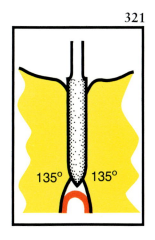

321

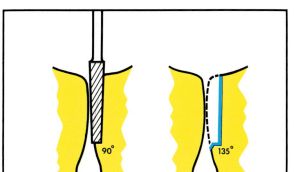

322

the tip of the bur remains outside the tooth (**319**). If the bur progresses too far an unacceptable margin of approximately 90° will result (**320**). When adjacent teeth are being prepared for full veneer crowns the touching interproximal surfaces may be prepared simultaneously (**321**).

When only a single crown is required however, the torpedo shaped bur cannot be used interproximally without risking damage to the adjacent tooth, unless of course there is interproximal spacing. To avoid such damage a delicate tapered diamond or tungsten bur should be used for the interproximal reduction (**322**, left and **323**), and the adjacent tooth can be given some protection by the application of a metal matrix band. During this procedure it is advisable to look intently at the adjacent tooth that is to be avoided rather than at the tooth being prepared.

The shoulder resulting from the use of a tapered fissure bur will require bevelling (**322**, right) and this can be applied with a Baker-Curson bur slightly angled to the line of withdrawal (**324**).

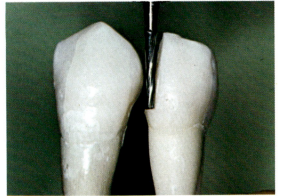

323

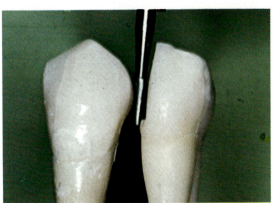

324

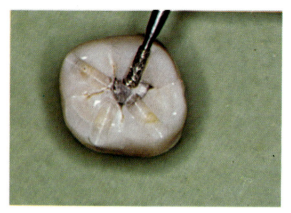

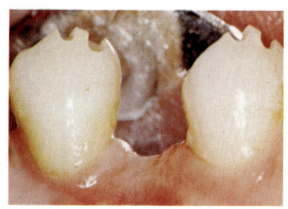

325, 326 The occlusal surface of a tooth being crowned will need to be reduced to provide room for coverage without interference from the opposing teeth. The room required is 0.75–1.0mm for metal alone. Sometimes all or part of this clearance already exists and so allowance must be made for this. In order to achieve the correct reduction it is helpful to cut a series of channels with a bur of known diameter to mark the depth of clearance required (**325**). The effectiveness of these channels can be appreciated by this buccal view (**326**).

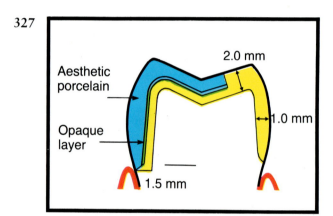

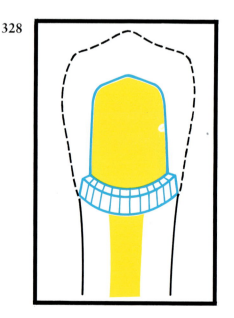

327, 328 If a metallo-ceramic crown is to be provided, tooth reduction has to be increased to 1.5mm in the areas concerned to make room for both metal and porcelain.

A minimum thickness of 0.5mm is required for the bonding alloy substructure. If the metal is in thinner section it may flex in use and cause the porcelain to crack. Also, if the alloy is too thin, it may sag in the porcelain furnace and thus distort. For the porcelain a minimum thickness of 1.0mm has to be allowed to mask the metal and achieve adequate translucency. These requirements therefore demand a shoulder width of 1.5mm wherever metal and porcelain is required (**327**, left). The marginal finishing line may be a butt-joint as shown here, which is acceptable as the bonding alloy is too hard to allow burnishing. Many operators,however, prefer a bevel to provide the bonded crown with 'ferrule' type support for the root, particularly if the tooth has been weakened by root canal therapy (**328**). With modern materials it is possible to cover the metal bevel with porcelain right to this margin.

Where porcelain coverage is not required, often palatally and lingually, reduction is required only to accommodate the metal, as in a standard full veneer crown, and a 135° chamfer margin is appropriate (**327**, right).

94

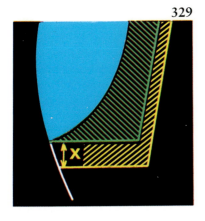
329

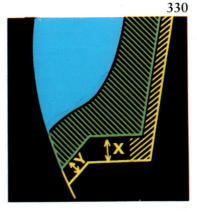
330

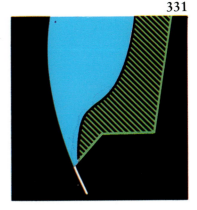
331

329–331 The options of marginal finish for bonded crowns can best be illustrated diagrammatically. The butt-joint shoulder preparation gives no support to the underlying tooth and results in the thickest cement lute at the margin (x). Bevelling of the margin (**330**) provides 'ferrule' type support for the tooth and results in a thinner cement lute (y). The appearance of the metal substructure at the cervical margin, as in **330**, may not be acceptable to the patient. If this is the case a skilled technician using modern materials should be able to disguise it by carrying the porcelain facing right to the edge of the restoration (**331**).

332 If aesthetic considerations apply to a posterior tooth and the patient objects to showing amalgam or gold there is the alternative of an inlay constructed in either porcelain or composite. This might well be preferable to the tooth destruction that goes with a full coverage bonded porcelain crown and it can give a comparable aesthetically pleasing result.

The cavity for such an inlay would need to satisfy the usual requirements of withdrawal form and the near parallelism of retention form which apply to any inlay cavity but without the bevelled margins.

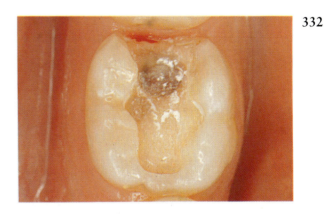
332

333 A base of glass ionomer will provide pulpal protection and its adhesion to sound dentine, as well as to composite, will aid in retention for a composite inlay.

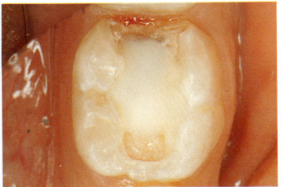
333

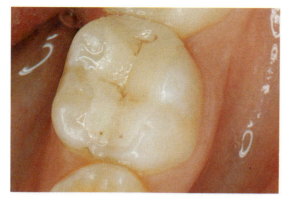

334 This example demonstrates the result that can be achieved by a porcelain inlay. A similar but monochrome effect can be obtained with composite inlays cured in the laboratory. Both types are cemented with composite cements. The big advantage of these inlays over posterior composite fillings is that the problems of curing shrinkage are overcome, i.e., the loss of marginal integrity and the fracturing of marginal enamel. Contact points may also be more effectively reproduced with indirect composite inlays than by the direct technique. Indirect restorations are also harder and resist wear to a much greater extent.

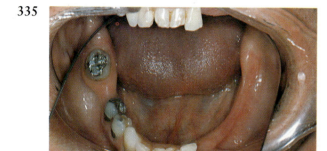

335 Whenever a full veneer crown or crowns are required in association with the provision of a partial denture, as here in the case of the lower right second premolar and third molar, it is important to anticipate the partial denture design before the crowns are made. Apart from the need to make the crowns before the denture, as it is unnecessarily complex to have to make a crown to fit within an existing prosthesis, there is always the possibility that the external design of the crown may well assist the retention of the denture. At the very least it should not impede the denture design by the introduction of unwanted undercuts.

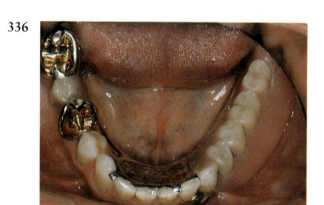

336 It will be seen that the gold crowns have been made with rest seats and their circumferences have been provided with just enough bulbosity to give the right amount of undercut for the retentive clasp arms.

In other designs the denture may include a cobalt chrome baseplate which requires the lingual and interproximal aspects of crowns to create precise guide planes to aid the stability and retention of the denture.

13 Anterior veneers

Although many aesthetic defects in anterior teeth can be remedied by acid-etch composite techniques, such restorations do not remain in good condition for more than a few years. This is due to the tendency of a composite restoration to stain, particularly at the margins, and to wear if placed in a vulnerable area. These defects can, admittedly, be repaired from time to time by skimming off the affected parts and resurfacing with an addition of new composite material. They are therefore quite appropriate as semipermanent restorations particularly in young people if the gingival margin has not yet assumed its mature position. However for a more permanent solution a veneer or crown should be considered.

A crown will be the choice if there is considerable loss of tooth tissue (see Chapter 14) either due to extensive mesial and distal caries or a fracture that extends over the palatal or lingual surface. If however the defect is confined to the labial surface and an improvement of appearance rather than treatment of dental disease is required, then a veneer can be considered. This will have several advantages over a crown, such as minimal tooth preparation without the need for local anaesthesia, ease of impression taking and preservation of the palatal surface thus avoiding any problems with occlusion. Veneers do however require a technician with special ceramic skills and they also take more time at the chairside to fit. This time factor is however offset by time saved at the preparation stage.

Custom made veneers can be constructed from composite or porcelain, both being made in the laboratory and cured or fired in the appropriate oven or furnace. The best results in terms of resistance to wear, aesthetics and cleansability are obtained from ceramic or porcelain veneers.

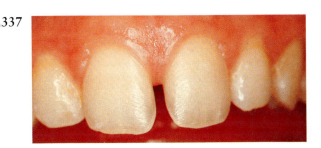
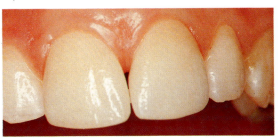

337, 338 A patient's insistence on the elimination of a diastema between two perfectly sound teeth presents an ideal opportunity to use ceramic veneers. Almost total preservation of the teeth is possible with only minimal interference required to achieve a most pleasing result.

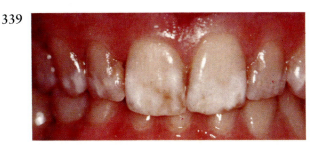
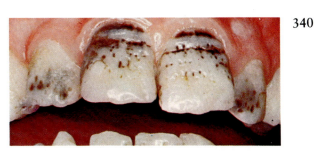

339, 340 Similarly where hypoplasia has disfigured otherwise intact crowns a welcome improvement in appearance can very readily be achieved with veneers.

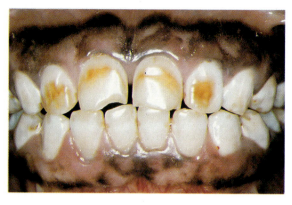
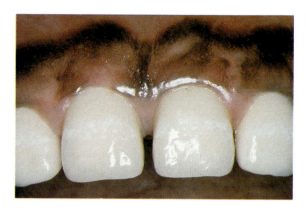

341, 342 These upper incisors are also badly disfigured by enamel hypoplasia (**341**) but this is confined to the labial surfaces. In all other respects the teeth are quite sound.

Placement of porcelain veneers (**342**) has made a dramatic improvement to the appearance both in terms of colour and shape. In this instance it was the patient's wish to maintain the central diastema but this could easily have been closed if preferred.

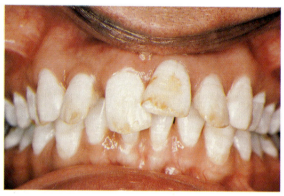
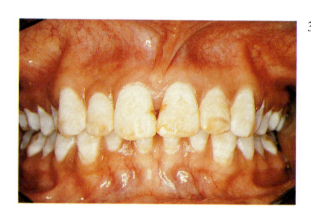

343–346 The hypoplasia of the upper incisors of this patient was further complicated by irregularity of the teeth (**343**). A plan was required which combined orthodontic and restorative treatment.

Orthodontic treatment was completed first (**344**). Porcelain veneers were then fitted to all four upper incisors and the canines (**345**). Stability was maintained by the use of composite retained splints fitted palatally to the canine and the two incisors at each side (**346**).

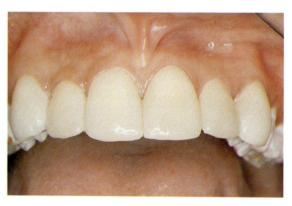
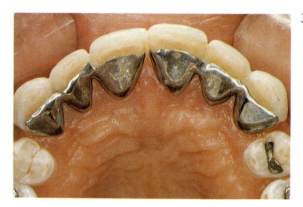

347 This severe combination of erosion and abrasion has exposed a considerable amount of dentine which may well be severely irritated by the cementing composite used with the porcelain veneers. Furthermore the amount of enamel available for retention has been greatly reduced. Both these problems can be overcome by applying glass ionomer to the exposed dentine before taking impressions. This will protect the dentine from the composite and will bond to the dentine. The composite in its turn will readily bond to the glass ionomer.

It is advisable to apply glass ionomer to any dentine inadvertently exposed during tooth preparation for veneers otherwise afterpain may occur which can be severe.

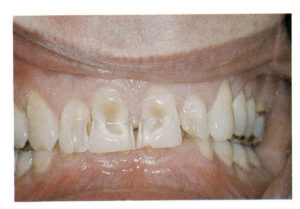

The veneering technique

A considerable surface of enamel is needed if good retention for the veneers is to be obtained by composite using the acid-etch technique. It is possible to place veneers without any preparation of enamel other than cleaning and etching and if the teeth are intact then enamel will be available in abundance. This will, of course, lead to the labial surfaces being considerably more prominent than previously but if, for instance, all upper front six teeth are veneered this prominence may not be obvious. If only a single tooth in a regular arch requires veneering, this approach may not be acceptable.

There are several reasons for undertaking some tooth preparation prior to veneering, whether single or multiple veneers, though, as has already been stated, involvement of dentine is to be avoided. This is not only because it will reduce the amount of available enamel, but because it can result in pulpal irritation and pain.

Firstly, a general reduction of the labial enamel will create room to inset the veneer and keep the prominence of the labial surface to a minimum. This is not only of importance for the single upper incisor but also for any lower incisors where these are in close proximity to the palatal surfaces of the upper teeth.

Secondly, several advantages accrue from the creation of a definitive finishing line around the perimeter of the surface to be veneered. To the technician it identifies the boundaries of the veneer, whilst for the clinician it will define the area that requires etching and, when the veneer is being fitted, it will provide positive location. This latter point is particularly relevant when multiple veneers are being placed. Without each locating to its intended position there is the risk that one veneer will encroach on the space required for its neighbour.

A further advantage is that preparation of the enamel will ensure that prismatic and not amorphous enamel is presented to the etchant for the creation of adequate micropores.

348, 349 Mesial and distal channels (**348**) can readily be cut with a bullet shaped or small round diamond bur without risk of involving dentine.

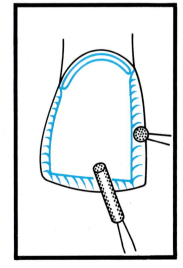

348

349

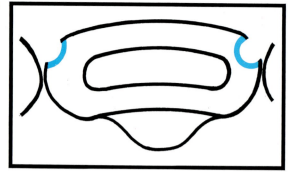

These channels should be made without undercuts (**349**, left) and kept clear of the adjacent teeth. Remembering the line of insertion for a veneer is from a labial direction it will be seen that the right hand groove in **349** has created an undercut. Any attempt to seat the delicate porcelain veneer in such a situation is to risk breaking it.

A groove in the gingival region must be placed with extreme delicacy if dentine exposure is to be avoided. This is because the enamel is becoming very thin here and if the veneer is to approach the amelo-cemental junction it is perhaps wise to omit this groove altogether.

Depending on the incisal relationship with the opposing teeth an incisal bevel may be added to the preparation (**348**). If incisal coverage by porcelain can be tolerated, such a bevel will allow protection of the composite joint, will look more pleasing and will assist greatly in correct location when fitting the veneer. When the periphery has been defined the enamel within it can be reduced.

350 This cross sectional diagram shows the delicate nature of the gingival groove, the space created for insetting the veneer and the direction of the incisal bevel.

350

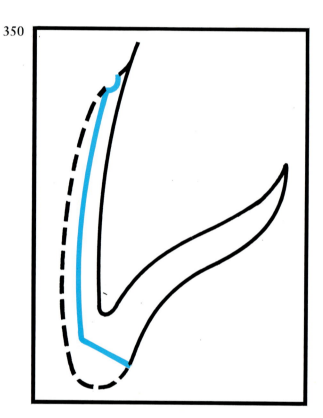

351

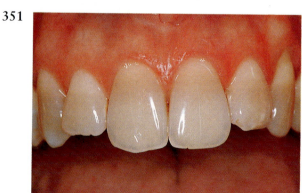

351 A comparison of the gingival quarter of these teeth with the remainder of the labial surfaces reveals disfiguring discolouration from the misuse of tetracycline during the time of their formation.

352 The labial surfaces and incisal tips have been reduced as described in **348**. A silicone impression of the upper arch is taken and an alginate impression of the lower. After noting the shade and any particular characteristics of the teeth requiring reproduction in the veneers the patient is dismissed. Temporary dressings of the prepared teeth are not required or even feasible.

When the veneers have been constructed the fitting surfaces need appropriate treatment to ensure the retention of composite resin to the porcelain.This is achieved either by sandblasting or etching the fitting surface by the technician. This can be further aided by the application of a silane coupling agent. It is wise to have the technician protect this surface from contamination, by handling or by saliva at try-in, with a thin layer of unfilled resin applied with a small brush and polymerised with a 15 second exposure to the curing light.

353 The first step in fitting veneers is to clean the tooth surface of any debris or plaque with a non-fluoride containing polishing paste or a mixture of pumice and water. Etchant in coloured gel form is then applied to the prepared surfaces. Adjacent teeth are protected with a celluloid strip or, more conveniently, by dead soft matrix strip which stays where it is placed (e.g. Conform, Westone Products Ltd, London W1M 5FU).

354 The gel is thoroughly washed off, the tooth dried and the enamel examined for a frosted surface which will indicate that satisfactory etching has been achieved. From this stage on the newly etched surface must be protected from any contamination with water or saliva. If this occurs a further 15 seconds of etching will be required.

355 Complete but not excessive coverage of the fitting surface of the veneer with composite resin is assisted with a miniature brush whilst the veneer is steadied by a plastic instrument. It is important to ensure that the margins are not starved of composite which might result in marginal voids. On the other hand an excess of material will have to be removed creating unnecessary difficulties especially after curing.

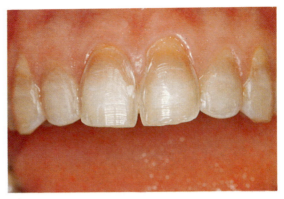

352

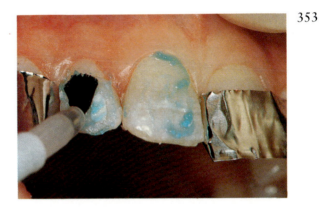

353

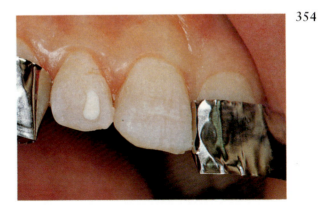

354

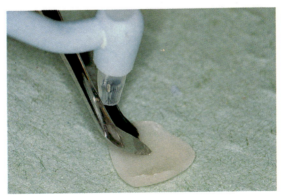

355

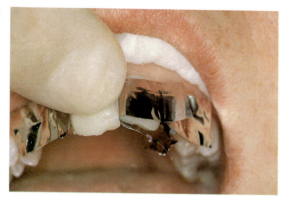

356 The tooth concerned is isolated from its neighbours with foil to prevent composite passing interproximally and the veneer is 'puddled' into place until it seats into the marginal grooves and the incisal bevel. This should not be rushed as too much pressure before the excess has had a chance to escape risks cracking the thin porcelain.

A short application of the curing light will tack down the veneer without fully polymerising the composite. This will ease the removal of gross excess and full polymerisation can then be achieved without the fingers obstructing the curing light.

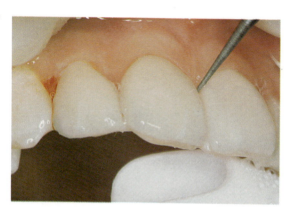

357 Excess composite and positive porcelain margins can be removed from around the veneer with a fine, so-called 'polishing', diamond of 10-15 micron grit size. Composite finishing strips may be used interproximally and a final polish given to any composite or porcelain so reduced with a polishing paste containing sub-micron particles of diamond.

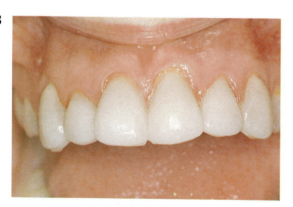

358, 359 The completed veneers and a happy patient.

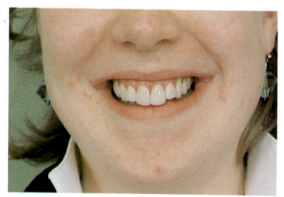

14 Anterior crowns

Anterior crowns are commonly made of porcelain, usually of strong aluminous porcelain with a central aluminous core for maximum strength. In situations of considerable occlusal stress the porcelain crown may be further strengthened by the use of a double platinum foil technique, the so-called McLean Sced technique (McLean and Sced, 1976), in which the outer foil, which has been tin plated, is left in the crown when it is fitted. The tin-plating of the foil allows the ceramic to bond to it and it is this bonding which resists the formation and propagation of cracks at the fitting surface which are claimed by McLean to be the cause of many broken crowns. If an even stronger crown proves necessary then it may be made of a metal substructure with porcelain fused to those surfaces that would otherwise be aesthetically unacceptable.

The use of jacket crowns

360 Extensive recurrent caries round large restorations is an indication for protection against further caries by full coverage with jacket crowns. Such restorations will also provide a most aesthetically acceptable result particularly when hypoplasia adds to the problem of caries, as here.

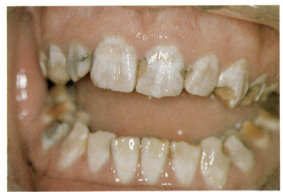
360

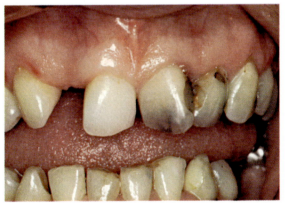
361

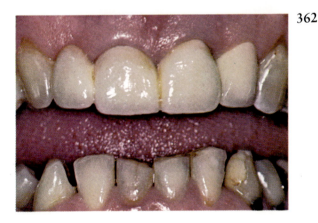
362

361, 362 The disfigurement resulting from the combination of large discoloured restorations in the upper left central and lateral incisors and the rotated central incisors (361) can be remedied with jacket crowns. In this case however a further improvement was made by including the missing upper right lateral incisor as the pontic to an all porcelain bridge fitted to the centrals. The left lateral incisor was restored separately with a porcelain jacket crown (362).

363

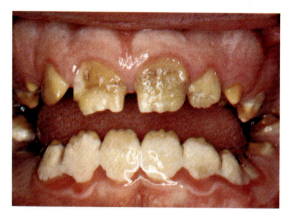

364

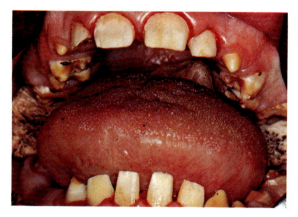

365

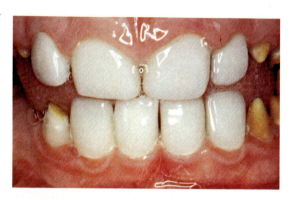

366

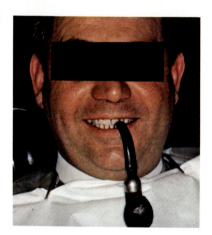

363–365 In this example of amelogenesis imperfecta the enamel is hypocalcified. As a consequence the teeth are misshapen and their rough surfaces are contributing to the heavy plaque and calculus deposits, especially around the lower incisors (**363**). After cleaning and establishing good plaque control, the upper and lower incisor teeth are prepared for shoulderless jacket crowns; because of the large pulps in such young teeth, only minimal tooth preparation is required (**364**).

The transformation in appearance following the fitting of eight jacket crowns (**365**) is likely to have a marked effect on the personality of the patient and their attitude to dental care, which fully justifies the use of advanced restorative work in so young a patient. It will of course be necessary to remake the crowns with normal shouldered preparations when the pulps have receded and the gingival contours matured.

366–368 Abrasion facets have been worn incisally by this patient's pipe on the left incisors and canines (**366**, **367**). The three jacket crowns have restored the appearance and have been characterised with cervical stain to blend in with his natural teeth (**368**).

367

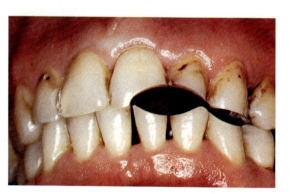

368

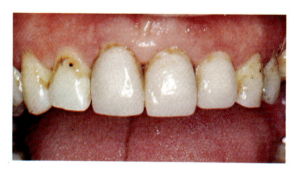

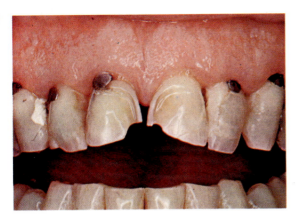

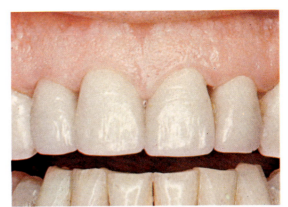

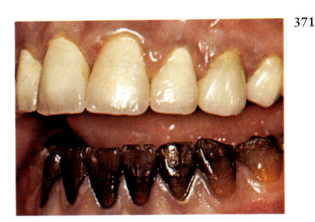

369, 370 In this example of erosion, labial enamel has been lost from the upper incisors (**369**) due to the acid environment in which the patient worked. A good aesthetic result has been obtained with four porcelain jacket crowns (**370**).

371 A dramatic improvement in appearance in this example of tetracycline staining can be achieved with multiple jacket crowns as can be seen at this halfway stage of the treatment.

372, 373 The space left by the early loss of the upper right lateral incisor has partially closed (**372**) leaving insufficient room for a partial denture to give a pleasing result. The space and the rather pointed and noticeable canine can both be dealt with by crowning to simulate a lateral (**373**). The 'lateral' shown here has had to be made with a tilted long axis and is inevitably rather wider than the contralateral tooth. However, in purely social terms the improvement in appearance is very acceptable.

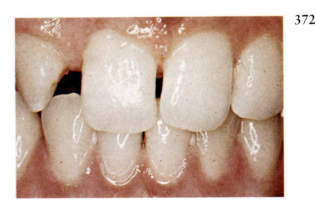

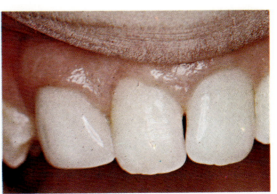

374

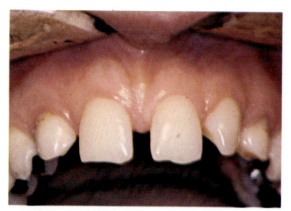

375

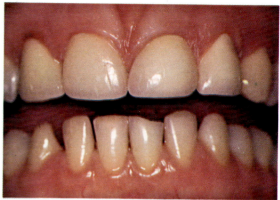

376

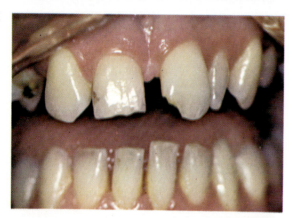

377

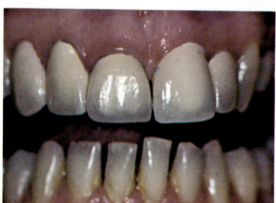

378

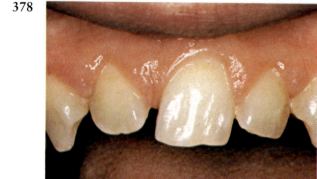

374, 375 The appearance resulting from missing upper lateral incisors and a retained primary canine (374) can be improved by four jacket crowns. An attempt has been made to disguise the width of the two central crowns by making the labial contour more convex than would normally be the case (375). The crowning of the primary tooth can be justified if the tooth is firm and there is no resorption of its root. However, the disparity in shape between the original primary tooth and that of the tooth being simulated makes it difficult to achieve a perfect cervical adaptation with consequent problems of plaque control. The marginal gingivitis apparent here will need careful home treatment by the patient.

376, 377 The unsightly appearance of these upper front teeth (376) is due to a number of circumstances including a missing lateral incisor, drift of a canine, fracture of a central incisor and presence of a 'peg' lateral incisor.

Jacket crowns have been placed on the upper left incisors and a simple cantilever bridge on the upper right central incisor and canine which fills the distal space with a simulated canine, whilst the natural canine is converted to look like a lateral (377). The aluminous core of the crown on the upper left central is visible and this should have been masked by covering with a thicker layer of dentine porcelain. It is also possible that there was insufficient reduction of the bucco-incisal tip in the preparation to create space for the porcelain.

378, 379 Early loss of the upper right central incisor has allowed the lateral incisor to move into the space (378). Other teeth in the quadrant have also moved mesially.

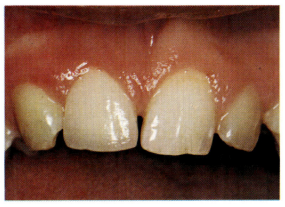

379

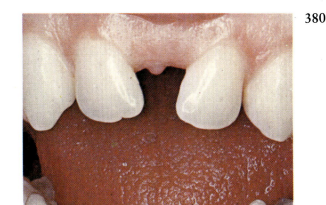

380

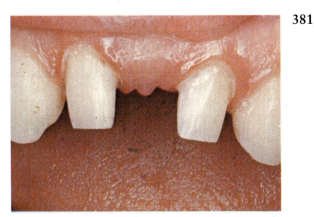

381

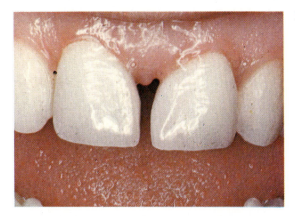

382

An acceptable appearance is created by crowning the lateral to simulate a central incisor and by grinding the tip of the canine to make it look more like a lateral incisor (379). Further improvement to the canine could have been achieved by adding a mesio-incisal corner with acid-etched composite.

380–382 At first sight, the tilting of the lateral incisors into the space from which the central incisors have been lost (380) suggests that jacket crown preparations would risk exposing the pulps. However, preparations were possible without resorting to post crowns (381). It is debatable whether the resulting jacket crowns (382) should have been made fractionally wider to avoid the diastema altogether.

383–385 The space due to the missing canine is only the width of half a tooth (383) making it impossible to fill it with a natural size canine. The space has therefore been partially filled with a jacket crown built out distally on the lateral. Looked at from the side with the lips retracted, it can be seen that the space has not been fully eliminated (384) although from the front the illusion is effective (385).

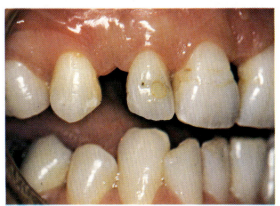

383

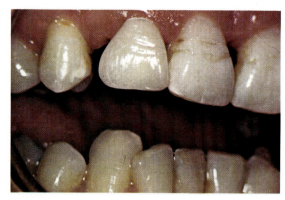

384

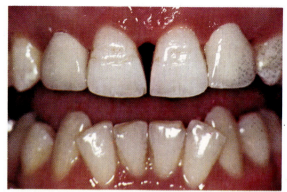

385

386–388 The left upper central incisor of this patient has erupted with its palatal surface facing labially (**386**). A standard jacket crown preparation is carried out (**387**) but the porcelain crown has been orientated to disguise the rotation (**388**). To improve the appearance further, the upper left canine requires some incisal grinding and the addition of acid-etched composite mesio-incisally to make it simulate the missing lateral incisor.

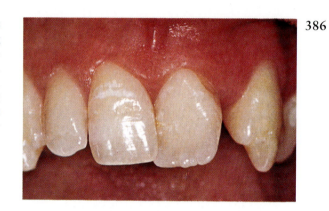

386

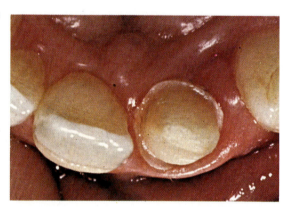

387

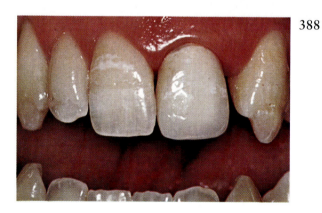

388

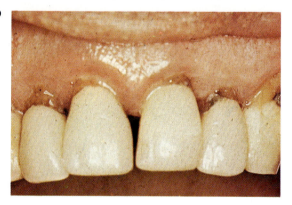

389

389–391 Gingival recession poses problems in anterior crown work, whether following the fitting of crowns as shown here (**389**), or in the natural dentition before crowns are contemplated. The narrowing of the root makes the establishment of 1mm shoulders in the preparation difficult if pulp exposure is to be avoided. There is also the aesthetic problem of not making the patient look 'long in the tooth'.

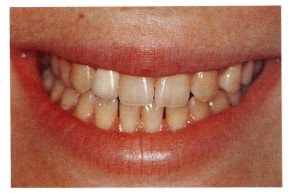

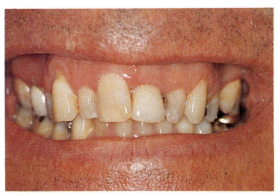

Whether this is a problem for the patient depends on their lip line. With a low lip line (**390**) he may not show the cervical portions of his crowns whereas with a high lip line (**391**) the cervical appearance may be of paramount importance.

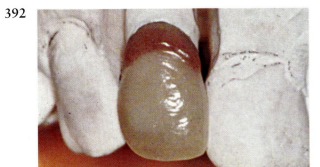

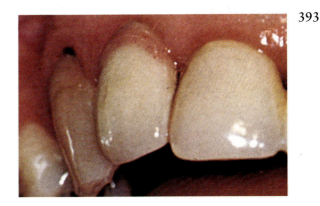

392, 393 This aesthetic problem can sometimes be solved by the use of pink porcelain to simulate gum, as in this lateral incisor.

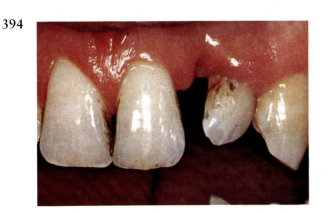

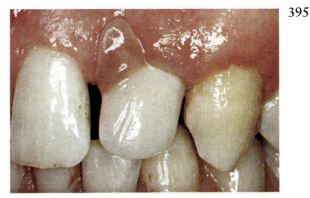

394, 395 The unsightly loss of alveolar bone due, in this case, to the removal of a supernumerary tooth from between the left central and lateral (**394**) can be made good by a projection of pink porcelain from the jacket crown made for the lateral incisor (**395**). The underside of the projection will need careful cleaning with dental floss.

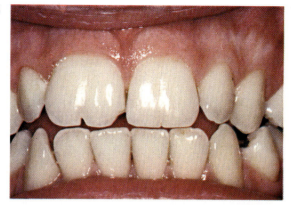

396 Not all disfigured teeth should be recommended for crowning. Apart from slight incisal notches and a small chip fractured from the mesial corner of the right central incisor, which can all be repaired with composite, these geminated upper central incisors are perfectly healthy, as are the supporting tissues. The best dental advice would be to persuade the patient to accept the excessive crown width. Extra wide crowns are rarely noticed, compared with anterior spacing which is instantly spotted by the general public. Correction of wide crowns is in any case difficult to achieve due to the wide cervical dimensions which cannot be reduced or disguised.

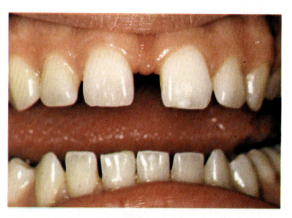

397, 398 This appearance of apparent microdontia (397) is probably due to the patient having jaws that are slightly larger than normal. The teeth and supporting structures are completely healthy and the problem is simply one of aesthetics. To show the patient what can be done, four acrylic jacket crowns can be made on a model of the upper jaws (398). These can then be used as temporary crowns if the patient wishes to proceed with porcelain jacket crowns. However, rather than put the gums and teeth at risk, it would be better not to interfere but persuade the patient to accept her appearance.

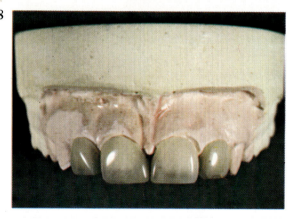

The use of post crowns

Sometimes it is inadvisable to attempt a jacket crown preparation because the amount of residual tooth tissue may be too little for satisfactory crown retention. A further contraindication to the provision of a jacket crown would be where the proclination, tilting or rotation of the tooth in question was so marked that the preparation was likely to result in pulpal exposure. It is also considered by many to be unwise to place a jacket crown on a non-vital tooth because of the increased brittleness of non-vital dentine and because of the loss of supporting dentine resulting from the access required for root canal therapy. In these and similar situations a post crown is the treatment of choice following placement of a suitable root filling. An exception to the latter argument would be when the pulp canal of the non-vital tooth has been obliterated with secondary dentine.

399 Ideally, a post-cum-core plus jacket crown design is chosen for any post crown situation. Should a new crown be required in the future, this allows one to be made without the need for removal of the post, a risky procedure.

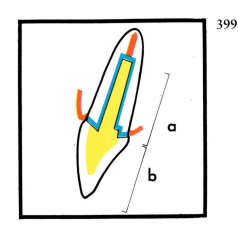

The post gains retention from the root of the tooth and the core simulates a jacket crown preparation to provide the retention for the crown. If the post/core is to be cast, the post hole must be cut with a slight taper for reasons of withdrawal and convenience form. However, such taper should be kept to a minimum if good retention is to be obtained and the root is not to be unnecessarily weakened. The length of the post should be at least the same as the crown it is to support (i.e. (a) = (b)) and preferably a little longer if the root allows.

400 The resulting cast post/core will have a slight protruberance at the coronal end of the post (arrowed) which fits into a matching 'anti-rotational notch' cut into the dentine thus resisting dislodgement of the post and core by rotary forces. When the post/core is cemented in place the core and the cervical shoulder of dentine resemble a jacket crown preparation and is treated as such for the construction of the crown.

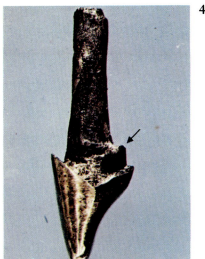

401 This series of grossly carious and misaligned upper incisors requires crowning both for reasons of restoration and appearance.

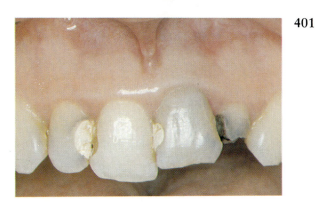

402 The resulting preparations vary according to how much sound tissue is left on each tooth. The upper right central incisor is vital with enough crown tissue to allow a jacket crown preparation. The upper right lateral, with the aid of some blocking out cement, has also been prepared for a jacket crown. Both upper left incisors however had so little crown tissue remaining that elective root canal filling was undertaken. By the insertion of posts and cores the situation was converted to one requiring a set of four jacket crowns. This approach overcomes the problem often met with multiple post crowns of taking impressions when the post holes are all at varying angles to each other.

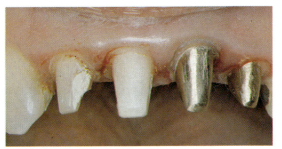

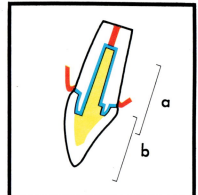

403 When the root of a tooth requiring a post crown is shorter than normal, as for instance following an apicectomy, it is possible to achieve the required post hole length by retaining coronal dentine and not reducing the natural crown to gum level. The dentine thus preserved can become part of the jacket core and effectively increases the available post hole length. The a/b ratio is therefore maintained.

404 This upper left lateral incisor has a short root resulting from periodontal disease which has lengthened the clinical crown. It has been possible to add to its effective length by preserving dentine in the core position.

405, 406 The post and core are shown here partially (**405**) and fully inserted (**406**). An added refinement to this technique has been to take the gold casting outside the core dentine. This supports the dentine and adds to the overall retention of the casting; it is a particular advantage when dealing with a small tooth where the access for root canal therapy and the partial jacket preparation has left the remaining tooth tissue rather weak.

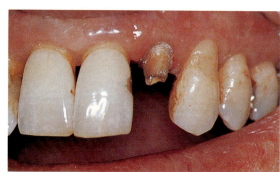

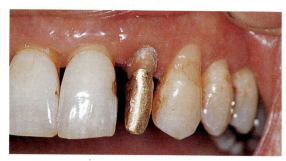

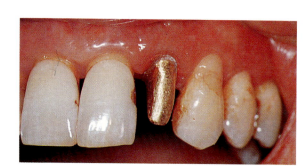

Prefabricated post systems

The cast post and core technique has universal application and can cope with elliptical root canals, overly wide canals and situations of excessive tooth loss which require a cast diaphragm to restore or support what is left of the tooth. The difficulty often associated with cast post crowns is that of taking a complete impression of a long and thin post hole. This difficulty can be overcome in one of two ways; by the use of a prefabricated post at the impression stage or by fitting a prefabricated post at the chairside. The latter solution, in effect, converts a post crown situation to a jacket crown

situation thereby eliminating the need for an impression of the canal and at the same time reducing laboratory costs. All prefabricated systems are limited to teeth with canal diameters that fall within the range of the posts provided.

Both prefabricated techniques reverse the approach to the post hole preparation. Whereas, in the traditional method of post construction, a post is made to fit whatever size and shape the posthole turns out to be, with the prefabricated technique, a posthole is cut to a predetermined size that will accept the chosen prefabricated post.

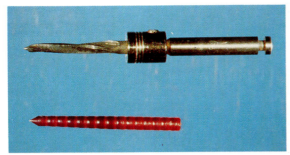

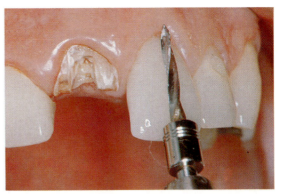

407 One prefabricated post system, an example of which is shown here, provides a series of six engine reamers of increasing diameter, with matching burnout plastic posts.

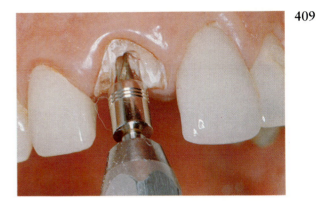

408 A sliding depth marker on the reamer can be fixed at the length required for the post hole. This length should be at least equal to the length of the intended crown and can be estimated by placing the reamer next to the contralateral tooth.

409, 410 The engine reamer creates a post hole of precise depth and diameter into which is introduced a matching plastic post.

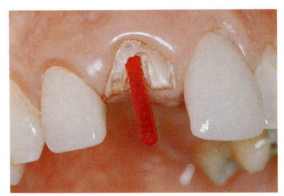

411 This may then be waxed up in the mouth in the form of a jacket crown preparation. After removal and casting it is cemented prior to impressions for a jacket crown. The plastic post is burnt out of the investment mould along with the blue wax prior to casting.

   If an indirect technique is preferred a smooth plastic post can be used in combination with an overall impression (see **480–483**) and the post/core, together with the crown, can be made in the laboratory.

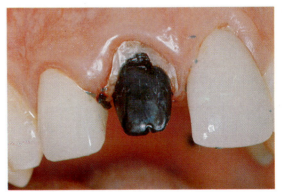

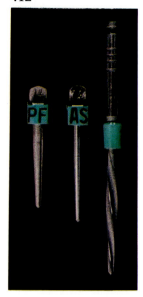
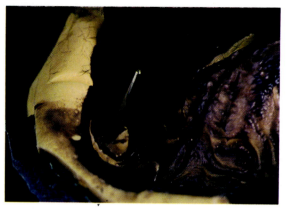
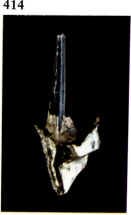

412–414 A similar approach to post crown design consists of casting the metal core onto the metal preformed post. This type of post serves to simplify the impression technique, as does the burnout post. As it is made of a high strength alloy often by a wrought rather than cast method, it is much stronger than cast gold and is preferred if it is thought that thin posts might distort in use (see **449**).

One such system is described by Mooser (1970). Matching posts and reamers (**412**) are provided in a range of sizes (Metaux Precieux SA) with the posts being of base metal (AS) and precious metal (PF).

The post hole is shaped precisely with the engine reamer and made slightly elliptical at the outer end for anti-rotational reasons. The base metal post is inserted and an overall impression taken (**413**).

In the laboratory a precious metal post is substituted in the working model for the base metal post. A core is waxed round this post and cast onto it. Note how the core of yellow gold extends into the anti-rotational groove and the shoulder of the casting has been created in a diaphragm (**414**). Note also that the post of precious metal has a longitudinal vent to allow the escape of cement at the fitting stage.

Prefabricated post and core systems

The essential benefit of a prefabricated post with core attached is that a post crown situation can be converted to a jacket crown situation at the chairside. Thus any difficulties that may exist in relation to recording an impression of the post hole can be overcome.

In cases of multiple post crowns, if the post holes run at several different angles such difficulties can be insurmountable unless of course each crown is made separately.

Preformed posts and cores come in a number of types and designs but with the common theme - the post is fitted into a post hole which is precisely cut to accommodate it and the protruding core is then fashioned into a jacket crown shaped preparation.

The Charlton post is parallel-sided with a solid tapered core. A matching size post hole is cut with a bur and the post is cemented into this in a way comparable with the tailor made cast post. Resistance to rotation is provided by the flat sides given to the core which fit into a slot cut in the face of the root.

Other designs are based on a post with a screw thread incorporated. In the Kurer system a matching thread is cut in the dentine of the post hole with an engineer's tap. The core portion is cylindrical and solid with an 'occlusal' slot to allow the application of a screwdriver. Cement is introduced into the threaded post hole and the post/core is screwed home and trimmed to shape once the cement has set.

415–424 Representative of several more modern designs is the Radix Anker system, (Maillefer, CH-1338 Ballaigues, Switzerland). Its post (**415**), which is self-tapping, has several useful features. It is parallel-sided for maximum retention and safety and its thread is delicate but coarse pitched so as to create minimum stress when the thread is being cut. Vents running the full length of the post allow the egress of excess cement thus avoiding the build up of hydraulic pressure when fitting the post.

The apical third of the post is free of thread which gives positive location and the end is bevelled for easy insertion. The core is shaped to allow the application of a hand driver for screwing the post into the root canal. This then serves as a framework to retain composite resin which, after polymerisation, is prepared to take a jacket crown.

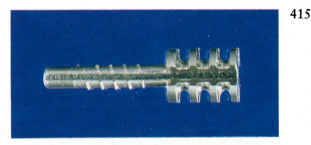
415

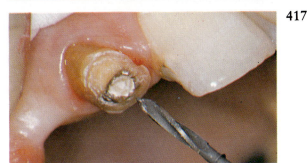
416

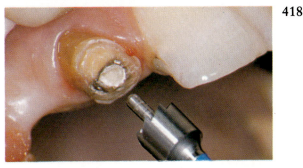
417

The kit of instruments (**416**) required for the insertion of a Radix Anker comprises, from left to right: an engine reamer to remove root filling material (**417**); a facing tool to flatten the face of the root to give a good fitting base for the core (**418**); a precision reamer to establish the exact dimensions required for the post hole (**419**); a blank post which mimics the actual post but without a thread (**420**); and a hand driver for inserting the post (**421**). The blank post allows a try-in to assess whether the post seats properly and gives the size, shape and position of core required. Shown beneath the post itself is a rotary paste filler which may be used to insert cement into the post hole.

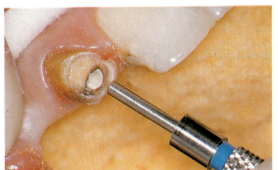
418

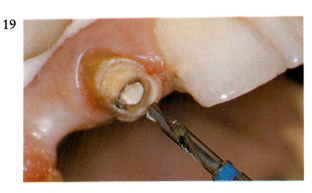
19

420

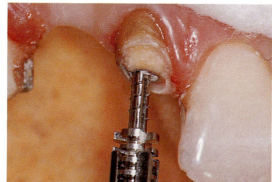

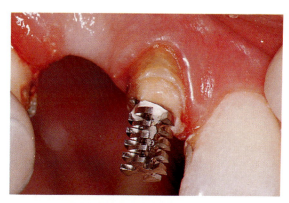

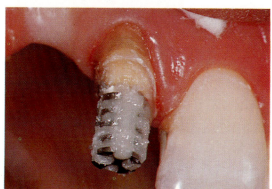

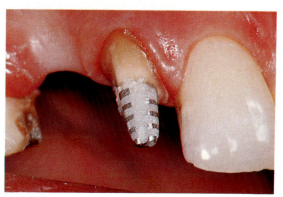

After the post is self-tapped into the root it is removed to allow the insertion of cement with a probe or paste filler after which it is re-inserted (**422**). Composite is adapted into the retentive core (**423**) and after polymerisation this is prepared to receive a jacket crown (**424**). Resistance to rotation is provided by introducing a small notch in the face of the root preparation at the top of the post hole and ensuring that some of the core composite resin is packed into this.

The Radix Anker system comes in two other forms. In one the core is of solid metal and tapered to provide a ready made core for use in premolar teeth. The core of the post, with little or no further preparation, is ready for the impression immediately after cementation without the need for the addition of composite resin. The other comes without a core but has a much longer post. Two or three of these can be inserted into the divergent root canals of a molar tooth and a core of amalgam or composite resin can be attached to the ends of the posts which protrude into the cavity.

Self-tapping and cemented posts give very good retention especially when a short root does not allow the traditional post hole length (see **403**). In such cases the length of the Radix post may require shortening.

Unlike the traditional cast system, no preformed post/core system is universally applicable. This is because they are available only in a limited range of sizes determined by the manufacturer and are mainly supplied with the post and core having a common straight line axis. Certain clinical features must exist therefore for one to be used satisfactorily: it must be possible to create a circular post hole in the root to accommodate the circular preformed post; and the root canal must be of a smaller diameter than the largest preformed post under consideration or it will be a loose fit and have poor retention.

If a very ovoid shaped root canal precludes the possibility of obtaining a circular post hole or if the axis of the core is required to be at a considerable angle to the axis of the post, (see **429**), then a cast post system will have to be considered.

Variations in post crown design

425, 426 In certain situations, such as marked palatal attrition or erosion (**425**), loss of space palatally may make it impossible to find room for the standard design of core and porcelain jacket crown. The problem may be overcome by the use of a bonded crown which needs less space for metal but if the situation is severe the only answer may be to cast post and core and then bond porcelain to this on the labial surface only (**426**). Should replacement be required at a later date this does mean the risky removal of the whole post crown.

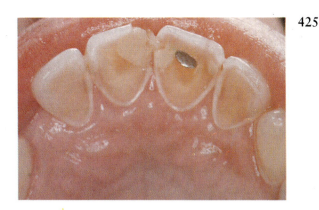

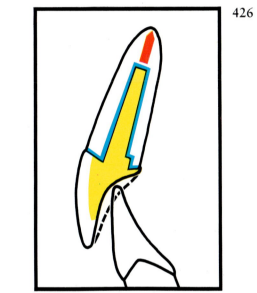

427 A problem sometimes encountered in a post crown preparation is the establishment of a good length post hole without deviating from the direction of the root canal which would risk an unwelcome undercut or worse, an accidental root perforation. Removal of gutta percha can be achieved safely with a Gates Glidden bur which has a blunt tip. The bur is driven up the canal by a combination of softening the gutta percha with frictional heat and cutting it with its blades. The blunt tip will guide the bur without risk of lateral perforation. Alternatively a slowly rotating round steel bur can be used but the progress of this must be checked frequently to ensure that the bur keeps on course and the gutta percha filling remains as the bull's eye of the target as it were. Transillumination of the root with a pen torch or fibre optic light can reassure the operator that this is the case.

428, 429 If an attempt is made to realign a proclined tooth into the arch it may be difficult to avoid a multiple traumatic exposure (**428**). Often the exposure can be predicted and an early decision made to perform an elective vital extirpation and root filling before restoring by means of a post crown. Realignment of crowns is possible using post crowns because it is not essential for the post and core to have a common long axis.

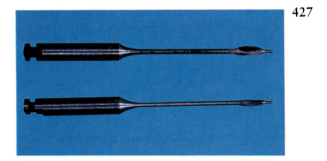

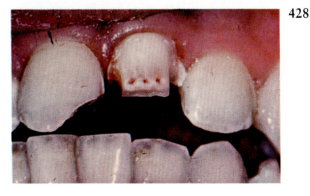

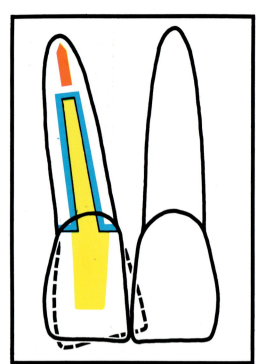

429

In this example of a mesially tilted central incisor (429) the core can be waxed up in a position quite independent of the long axis of the post. Thus an overlapping natural crown (dotted line) can be replaced with a jacket crown that is positioned regularly in the arch.

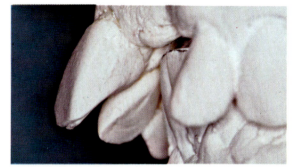

430

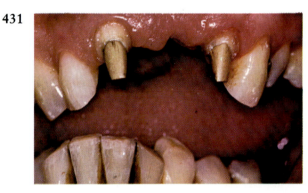

431

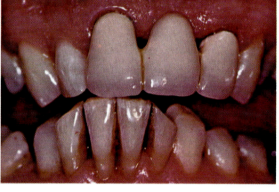

432

430–432 A partial denture for this patient (430) is inadvisable due to the lower incisors, even after having been ground to the line indicated on the study model, being too close to the palatal mucosa. Elective extirpation of the pulps and root filling of the upper right central and upper left lateral incisors allows posts to be fitted with their cores well positioned in the arch (431). Consequently both the missing tooth and the incisal protrusion have been remedied with an all porcelain bridge (432) based on jacket crown retainers.

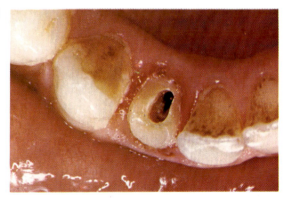

433

433–436 The fractured margin of the crown of the lower right lateral incisor is deeply subgingival on the lingual side (433) making it difficult to obtain the necessary butt-joint shoulder for a porcelain crown. This problem is overcome by constructing a cast post and core with diaphragm (434).

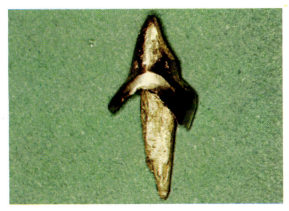

434

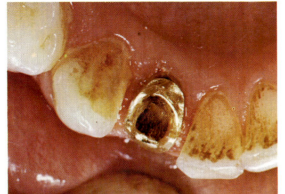

435

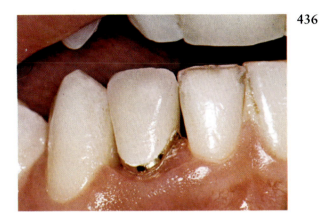

436

The cervical margin of the diaphragm has been closely adapted to the root by burnishing whilst its coronal surface provides the required shoulder for porcelain (**435**). In this example the diaphragm has been extended cervically to embrace the whole circumference of the root face to aid retention and resistance. It will also support the root from longitudinal fracture by the so-called 'ferrule' effect.

If the appearance of gold labially (**436**) is unacceptable the crown could alternatively be constructed of bonded porcelain. The ferrule effect would then be provided by the metal substructure of the crown with the labial margin of metal being hidden by porcelain.

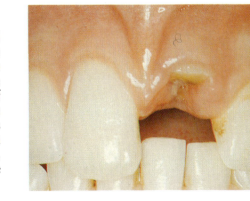

437

437–439 In this case the crown had been fractured well subgingivally thus creating considerable difficulties for crowning (**437**). It was decided to move the root orthodontically so that the root face was in an acceptable position for ease of preparation and impression. A hook of stainless steel wire was cemented into the root canal. This was connected by an elastic band to the labial arch wire of a removable orthodontic appliance (**438**). The resulting orthodontic movement produced the desired result (**439**).

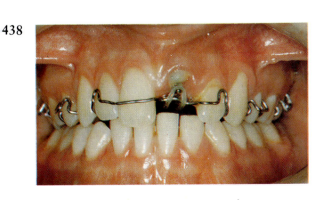

438

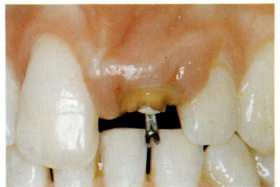

439

440

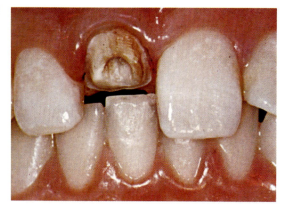

440–442 Here the lower incisors occlude so closely to the palatal aspect of the upper right central incisor which has been prepared for a post crown (**440**), that there is insufficient room for an adequate thickness of porcelain in the cervical region to resist fracture. A half diaphragm is included therefore on the casting to cover the cingulum area and to provide a shoulder (**441**) where there will be room to accommodate the porcelain without subjecting it to occlusal stresses from the opposing teeth (**442**).

441

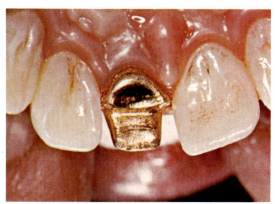

44

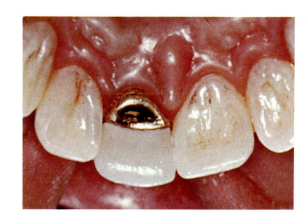

443

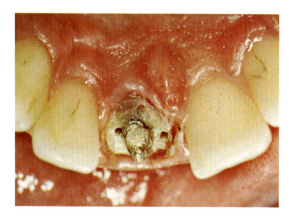

443, 444 Occasionally bizarre situations demand improvisation to provide a satisfactory result. In this situation (**443**) for instance the core is inadequate to allow attempted removal of the post without risking the separation of core from post. The solution has been to cast a new core to fit over the old using a number of pinholes cut in the dentine for retention as for a pinlay (**444**).

Porcelain crown characterisation

444

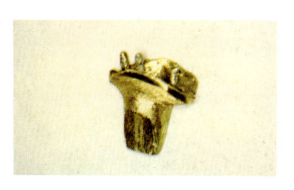

Aesthetics in relation to porcelain crowns is an art and whole books are devoted exclusively to the subject. Consequently the subject is covered only briefly in this book. A crown should blend imperceptibly with the adjacent teeth, rather than represent the technician's concept of the ideal. A clear prescription should be sent from chairside to laboratory and this sometimes results in the use of stains which, when judged in the laboratory, seem to disfigure the crown but when seen in the mouth look perfectly harmonious (see **368**).

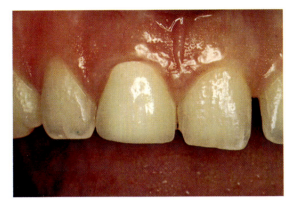

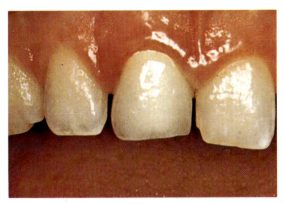

445, 446 The porcelain crown for the upper right central incisor is perfectly sound from a technical and biological point of view. However it has been made without consideration for the appearance of the natural teeth which surround it (**445**). The shade is wrong, lacking any gradation in colour such as that displayed by the contralateral tooth. Its shape is that of a stereotype central incisor rather than mimicking its partner. The contact points have been closed which is wrong for this patient. The remake crown deals with all these points and results in a pleasing natural appearance (**446**).

447 In contrast to **445** the characterisation in shape of the porcelain crowns for the upper left incisors completely matches that of the natural contralateral teeth. Perhaps a little more white and orange stain, delicately applied, would have made the illusion complete.

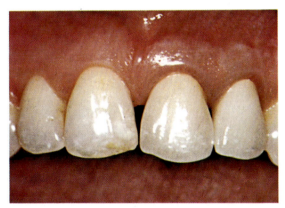

Some errors in post crowns

448, 449 The post crown on this upper right central incisor has become protruded (**448**) and after its removal, inspection showed that the post was too thin (**449**) for this particular situation. The heavy attrition of the lower teeth should have alerted the operator to the heavy forces that were likely to be applied to this crown. If it is inadvisable to widen the canal to increase the strength of a cast post then greater strength can be obtained by using a strong prefabricated wrought metal post.

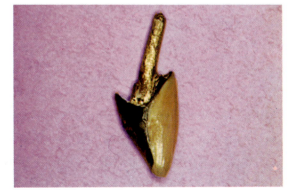

450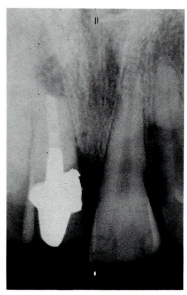

451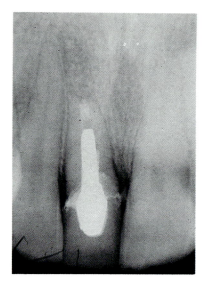

450, 451 The post crown on a traditional cast post (450) has become loose. However the original posthole was not long enough for sound retention and furthermore, what posthole there was had not been fully utilised. The remade crown (451) has a good length of near parallel post which should not be dislodged.

452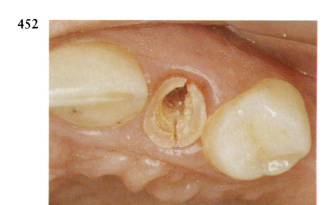

452 Too large a post hole will unduly weaken the supporting root. This is a common occurrence in a slender rooted upper lateral incisor with the risk of a longitudinal fracture as seen here. The fracture is not always as obvious as this but it should be searched for, perhaps aided by a disclosing solution (see 52) when a history is given of frequent loss and recementation of the post crown.

15 Impression techniques

Introduction

It is possible, though often time consuming, to fabricate patterns for gold restorations in the mouth (see **411**). This is known as the direct technique. Complex gold work, however, and all porcelain work has to be made in the laboratory, where the technician uses a replica of the patient's dentition. This is known as the indirect technique.

In order to replicate the patient's dentition, the technician requires impressions of the upper and lower arches. From these will be made, using special die stones and dental plaster or stone, a working die of the tooth or teeth to be restored, a working model to hold the die in the correct relationship to the adjacent teeth and an opposing model to indicate the occlusal relationship between the upper and lower teeth.

If the inlay, crown or bridge is to be successful, attention must be paid to precision and accuracy at all stages of its manufacture, starting at the chairside with accurate impressions and occlusal records. Particular accuracy is required for the impression of the arch containing the tooth to be restored. The working die is made from this impression out of hard and accurate stone which gives details of the surface of the tooth preparation which are crucial for the marginal fit of the restoration and its retention.

The die will be held within the model of the total arch and accuracy here will ensure that contact points of the restoration with adjacent teeth are adequate and correctly shaped.

The opposing model will give the information required to construct the restoration with an occlusal surface which is fully functional but without interferences either in initial contact or in lateral and protrusive excursions. To enable it to do this an occlusal record is required which gives the relationship of the upper and lower arches to each other. For single straightforward restorations a simple wax occlusal record or a functionally generated pathway record (FGP) may be sufficient. For complex work more sophisticated information will be required to allow the working and opposing models to be mounted on an articulator which is capable of reproducing the patient's jaw movements.

Developments over the last decade have given the profession a wide choice of elastomeric impression materials which are both accurate and easy to use. These rubbers have largely superseded other materials, such as composition and alginate, formerly used in the construction of indirect restorations, whilst reversible hydrocolloids remain popular with some practitioners.

Silicone materials are probably the most commonly used elastomeric and most of these are provided in two viscosities, usually in contrasting colours; low viscosity for ease of introduction into all the minute detail of the prepared tooth and a higher viscosity to provide the bulk of the impression. These are often referred to respectively as perfecting paste and putty.

The various techniques by which impressions are taken with these materials are classified in Appendix 5, the choice of a specific material being left to the preference of the operator. Basically they are divided into one-stage or two-stage techniques with stock or special trays.

The one-stage technique involves mixing the putty and perfecting paste simultaneously. Once mixed, the putty is placed in the tray and is coated with the paste. After insertion into the mouth they set together. This technique is thus slightly quicker than the two-stage but requires chairside assistance and does not always reproduce marginal detail of the preparation with sufficient accuracy. To improve this it is often necessary to load some of the paste into a syringe and to inject it around the prepared tooth before insertion of the loaded impression tray.

The two-stage technique starts with an impression in putty alone to which perfecting paste is added prior to it being re-seated for the final impression. This approach doubles the time taken for the impression material to set but can be used by the single-handed operator and more easily records the necessary marginal detail. The need for injecting paste round the prepared tooth is eliminated as the set putty ensures that the paste is well adapted to the preparation margins. This can offset, to some extent, the time needed to allow both stages to set.

A rigid stock tray is the tray of choice unless the shape of the patient's dentition does not fall within the range of available trays. A special tray may sometimes be preferred for particularly complex or extensive work.

Gingival retraction

For periodontal health, the gingival margins of all prepared teeth should finish ideally in a supragingival position. This has the added benefit of making them easily seen and accessible without causing gingival trauma. Impressions can then be taken without interference of gingivae or blood.

Often however, caries extends sub-gingivally so that after preparation the margin is below gum level. Sub-gingival preparation may also be necessary in order to gain sufficient length of preparation for adequate retention, especially where a tooth has a short clinical crown. In either case the advantages outlined may be regained by local gingival surgery to remove gum tissue thereby restoring the margin to a supragingival position (see **174, 295**).

It may not always be appropriate, however, to remove the gingival tissue, for example where the gingival margin has required placement subgingivally for aesthetic reasons. In such cases it is necessary to retract the gum temporarily in order to reveal the margin of the preparation whilst it is being recorded in the impression.

This is usually accomplished with a proprietary retraction cord, often supplied impregnated with adrenalin or an astringent, and sometimes further aided with an alum/adrenalin solution (see **119** and Appendix 3) when it proves particularly difficult to obtain a dry field. Dryness is crucial to success when using a hydrophobic impression material, such as a silicone, as the presence of saliva or blood will prevent it reaching the margins of the preparation. For this reason it is advisable to isolate well with cotton wool rolls which should be left in place throughout the impression procedure. To remove them just prior to inserting the impression tray is to risk wetting the area with the cheeks and tongue. The cotton wool rolls, which cannot easily be sterilised, should be cut from the impression before sending it to the laboratory to avoid cross infection. The impression, however, can readily be sterilised by immersion for one minute in a 1% solution of hypochlorite, after which it should be rinsed thoroughly in water.

453 Retraction cord is available in various thicknesses and, for the two-stage impression when the cord is left in place during the first stage, one should be chosen which is thick enough to hold the gingivae away from the tooth but not so thick that it covers up the margins it was intended to reveal. A plaited or braided cord is easier to handle than a twisted thread and this should be placed into the gingival crevice with the aid of a flat plastic instrument. A chairside assistant can follow the operator with a second plastic instrument holding the cord in place whilst the next section is being inserted.

Sufficient excess of cord should be left buccally to aid its rapid removal with tweezers just before the impression tray is inserted.

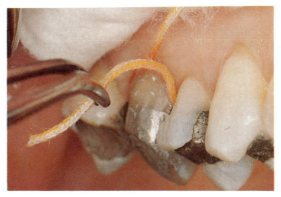

453

454 When the gingival crevice or pocket is deeper than the diameter of the cord, one turn of cord may not be sufficient to achieve satisfactory retraction of the gum. To wrap the cord a second time round the tooth would make it difficult to remove speedily. In this case a single turn of cord is fitted within the gingival crevice to be left there throughout the impression procedure whilst a separate thicker piece is placed on top, to be removed just prior to inserting the impression.

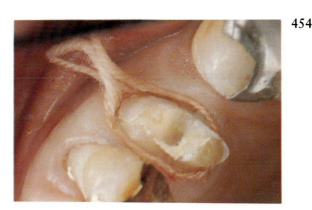

454

455, 456 The effect of the application of retraction cord can be seen in these 'before and after' pictures. The upper right canine and upper left central incisor have been prepared for jacket crown coverage (**455**). If the cord has been effective the gums, immediately after its removal, should be seen to be retracted so as to present the cavity margins to the impression material (**456**).

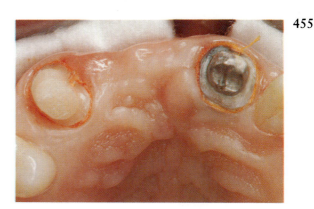

455

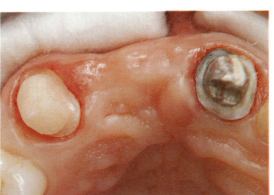

456

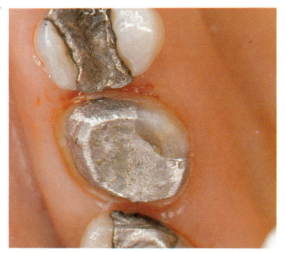

Single stage impression – stock tray

457 An impression is about to be taken of this upper first molar which has been prepared for a full veneer crown. The retraction cord has just been removed and the gingivae are seen to be satisfactorily everted to reveal the preparation's margins.

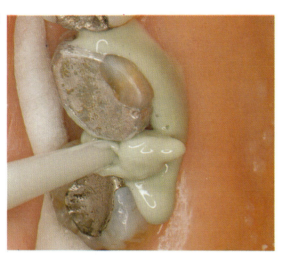

458 The silicone paste should be injected into the gingival crevice without delay. The whole of the tooth's prepared surface should then also be covered with the paste.

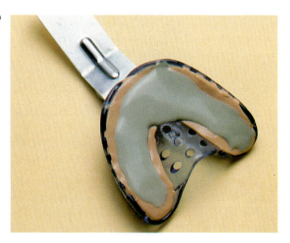

459 Meanwhile an assistant fills the stock tray with silicone putty and covers its surface with the remaining paste.

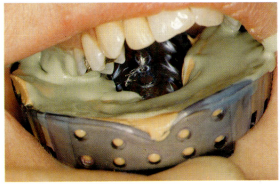

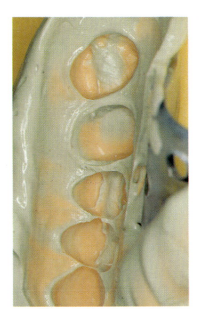

460 The tray is inserted over the teeth with firm pressure to ensure that the impression material reaches the furthest extent of the preparation. Pressure is then released and the tray held steady until the setting time recommended by the manufacturer has elapsed. The tray should be grasped firmly in the premolar region and snapped out of the mouth in a direction that matches the line of withdrawal for the preparation. The handle of the tray and a tilting action should not be used as this may distort the impression and reduce its accuracy.

461 The impression is then examined to confirm that all essential detail is satisfactorily recorded. This will include marginal definition of the preparation and the contact areas of the adjacent teeth. It can be seen here that the colour of the putty shows through the paste in many areas which indicates that the impression tray was well seated home.

Single stage impression – special tray

462, 463 In a stock tray the putty needs to be fairly viscous or it will run out of the tray when inserted and will not reach the depths of the prepared tooth. When a close fitting special tray is used, however, this is not a problem. The technique remains the same and the paste is injected as for a stock tray (462) but a much less viscous material may be used in the special tray, as can be seen here (463) from the fact that the paste has not been displaced to as great an extent as it would have been with a viscous putty.

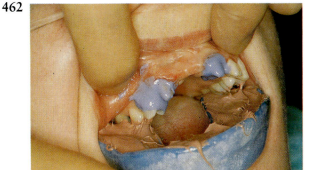

Two-stage impression – stock tray

Two advantages are claimed for the two-stage technique. Firstly, that an accurate putty impression, acting like a very close fitting special tray, will ensure that the perfecting paste is well adapted to the furthest reaches of the cavity margins. Secondly, that the effective setting shrinkage, that may occur with condensation cured silicone, is reduced to the minimum. Both putty and paste shrink on setting but most of the shrinkage takes place in the putty, as this constitutes the bulk of the impression material. If the putty is allowed to set before the final details are recorded by the paste, then the only setting shrinkage that might affect the accuracy of the final impression is that taking place in the very thin layer of perfecting paste.

For these benefits to be realised the first stage impression must be a full and complete one and the second stage impression must be fully inserted to ensure that the paste layer is made as thin as possible.

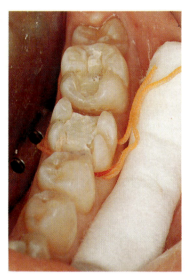

464

464 Moisture control is achieved and the retraction cord placed as before but with two variations applicable to the cord. The cord is left in place during the putty stage of the impression and considerable excess of cord is allowed to extend into the buccal sulcus.

Leaving the cord in place for the first stage keeps the gingivae retracted and enables the putty to take a good impression of the cavity margin, whilst the impression taken of the buccal excess of cord creates a channel in the putty. This channel is essential in order to allow escape of excess paste at the second stage. If it were not able to escape it would distort the putty by the hydraulic pressure created. If cord is not required, for instance when the cavity margins are supragingival, then channels will have to be cut in the putty impression with a scalpel.

465–469 The first stage impression is examined for completeness and freedom from air blows (**465**): once checked it is then prepared for the second stage. This entails removal of any nonessential parts of the putty that might impede its re-insertion. The interdental tags of putty, for instance, will not easily allow the impression to be re-seated and should be cut out either with a scalpel (**466**) and removed with tweezers (**467**) or, in one action, with Rongeur bone forceps (**468**).

465

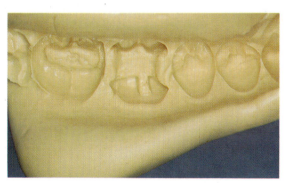

46

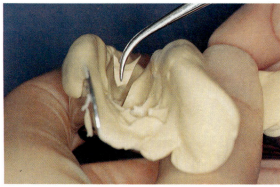

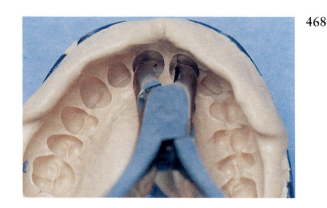

It is also wise to trim back the periphery of the impression (**469**). This is not required and only adds unwanted suction making the removal of the second stage more difficult. If the retraction cord came out with the first stage of the impression, it will be necessary to place another length in prior to the final impression.

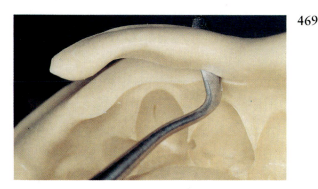

470, 471 The trimmed putty is given a good wash and is dried to present an uncontaminated surface to the wash of perfecting paste which is next applied (**470**). The impression is firmly seated after removing the retraction cord at the last possible moment. The heavy pressure of insertion ensures that the paste is 'injected' by the putty past the cavity margins and into the gingival crevice. Furthermore the paste layer is made as thin as possible to minimise the setting contraction.

Pressure must be relaxed immediately, before the paste sets, or there is the risk of elastic recoil occurring in the putty. This 'bounce', as it is sometimes called, is a result of compression of the putty, which recovers when the impression is removed and distorts the impression. The impression is inspected for completeness (**471**), particularly at the cavity margins, which is recognised by paste having entered the gingival crevices.

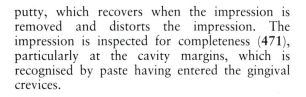

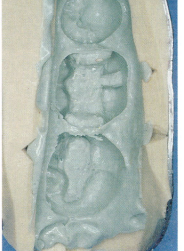

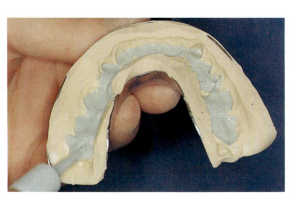

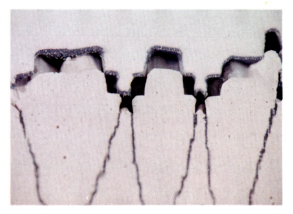

472 A sectional view of a poured model, with the impression slightly withdrawn and with the approximate root outlines pencilled in, demonstrates the successful retraction of the gingivae, the recording of the marginal detail and the thinness of the paste material.

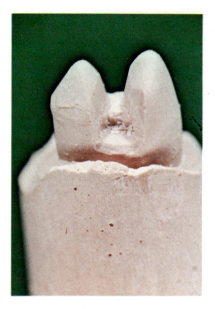

473 One of the dies separated from the model shows the clarity of marginal definition that can be achieved with a sound impression technique.

Impression technique with copings and special tray

474–479 If particular difficulty in recording marginal detail is experienced or anticipated, a technique with copings can be employed. This technique can also be an alternative to using an injection syringe with polysulphide rubber.

For these jacket crown preparations of the upper lateral incisor and canine (**474**) a preliminary impression is taken from which the technician pours a model on which to construct the copings (**475**). The copings are small 'impression trays' made individually in Duralay for each prepared tooth. At the same time an acrylic special tray is made which will accommodate the copings.

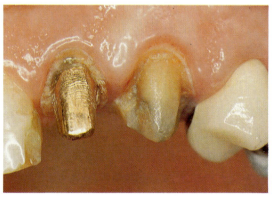

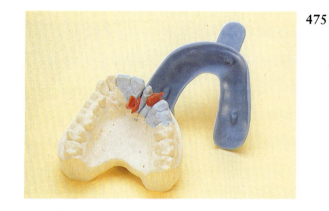

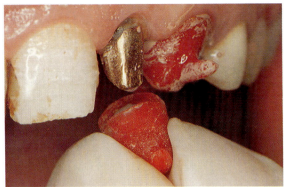

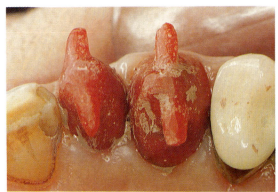

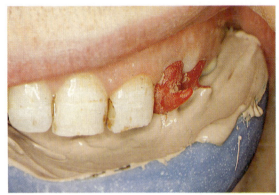

The copings are tried for accurate fit and can be refined, if necessary, with the addition of Duralay (Reliance Dental Mfg.Co., Worth, Ill., USA). After coating the inner surface with adhesive each coping is filled with light-bodied polysulphide impression paste and seated firmly onto its tooth (476, 477). It can be seen that each one has labial and palatal projections which secure the copings in the overall impression: the impression is taken with regular polysulphide using the special tray (478).

The resulting impression shows good reproduction of the margins of the prepared teeth (479).

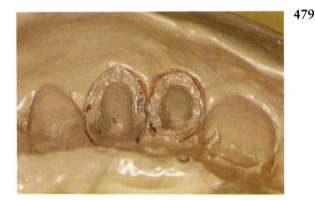

Anterior post crown impression technique

Introducing impression material into a post hole without trapping air can be difficult and the impression material can readily tear or distort. This problem can be overcome if the post hole is cut to a size and shape that will accept a preformed post (see Chapter 14).

480, 481 A plastic burnout post of the same dimensions as the prepared canal is placed and is used to record the post hole. Its outer end will have been flattened with a hot wax knife into a 'nailhead' and coated with adhesive to ensure that it stays firmly attached within the impression material (480).

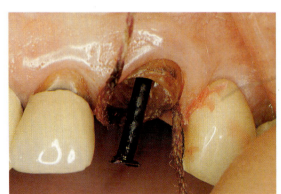

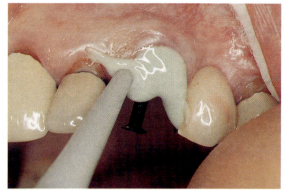

481

The gingival margin of the root face has been revealed with the aid of retraction cord and, following its slow removal with tweezers, the nozzle of a syringe injects silicone paste impression material into the gingival crevice (481) and subsequently over the plastic post.

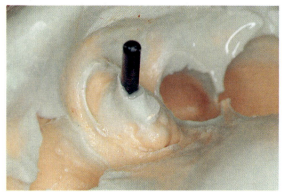

482

482 This is immediately followed by the insertion of a stock tray loaded with silicone putty surfaced with the remaining paste.

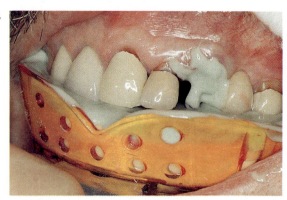

483

483 Care must be taken to withdraw the impression in the same direction as the axis of the post hole. The impression of the prepared tooth can be seen to be a combination of plastic post and silicone.

If uncertainty about the marginal definition exists a two-stage version of this technique can be used in which the plastic post is gripped within the first stage putty impression. Replacement of the putty impression for the second stage starts by placing the plastic post into its post hole. For this to be seen clearly it may be necessary to reduce the labial margin of the putty with a scalpel.

Recording occlusal relationships

If a patient requiring a single inlay or crown has a full complement of teeth whose cusps interdigitate positively, the technician may well be able to construct the restoration without any occlusal information other than that provided by the working jaw and opposing jaw models. Occlusal accuracy of the restoration can be judged by simply bringing the two models into the intercuspal position to check for absence of centric occlusal interferences, and by moving the models protrusively and laterally to confirm that interferences do not occur during such movements.

484 If there is any uncertainty in the dentist's mind that this can be done satisfactorily, an occlusal record should be made. In its simplest form this is produced from an arch-shaped sheet or double layer of pink wax suitably softened to record the cusps of the upper and lower teeth when the patient closes in the retruded arc of closure. This wax record can be refined by coating the indentations with a quick-setting temporary cement and asking the patient to close again in the retruded axis position. This will increase the accuracy with which the technician is able to locate his models whilst mounting them on a simple articulator.

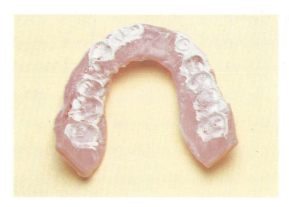

The functionally generated pathway (FGP)

If there is uncertainty about possible interferences during various jaw movements an FGP should be considered.

485–490 This simple but very effective occlusal record depends on defining and recording the space required, during function, by any of the teeth opposing the restoration which is to be constructed. Using this record the technician is able to create an occlusal surface for the restoration that does not intrude into this space thus avoiding interferences.

To define the space required the prepared tooth is covered with soft carding wax. For a posterior crown, retention for this wax is obtained by applying a tightly fitting copper ring (**485**). The ring should be trimmed so as not to damage the gums or interfere with the occlusion. Carding wax is next added to slight occlusal excess (**486**). The patient is then asked to close tightly into the intercuspal position and then, whilst keeping the teeth in close contact, to move into all possible lateral and protrusive positions. The wax is thus pushed out of the way of all opposing teeth (**487**). Any wax that has spread over the adjacent teeth should be removed. The functionally generated pathway is now ready to be recorded.

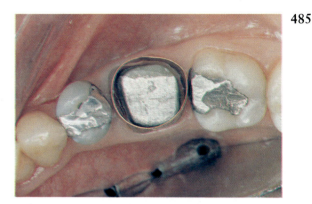

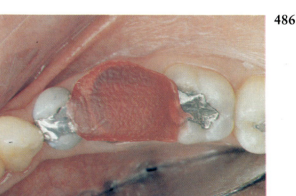

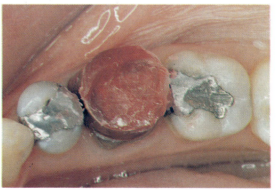

488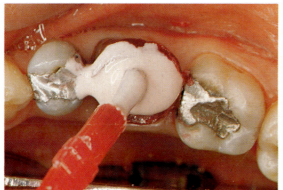

489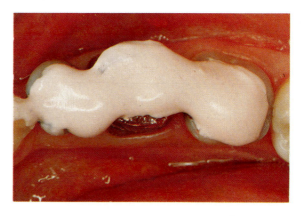

490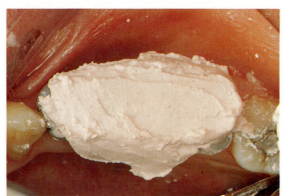

This is done with impression plaster which is quickly spread with a spatula or small brush (**488**) to cover both the wax surface and the occlusal surfaces of the two adjacent teeth (**489**), whilst it is still fluid enough to record the detail accurately. Further stiffer plaster is added to give a reasonable bulk (**490**) that will be strong enough to be handled in the laboratory.

The plaster record is used by the technician during the occlusal build up of the restoration to insure that it does not intrude into the space required for the opposing teeth. This is confirmed by showing that it is possible to place the plaster record close to the adjacent teeth without making contact with the wax or porcelain of the restoration.

Use of articulators

It is advisable to mount the patient's casts on an articulator in order to establish an accurate occlusal relationship for complex or multiple restorations. A semi-adjustable articulator, such as the Denar or Whipmix, will usually provide a satisfactory reproduction of the jaw movements, once set to various parameters for a particular patient.

The two main parameters are the relationship of the upper dental arch to the cranium and the lower arch to the upper arch when the jaw is in the retruded axis position.

491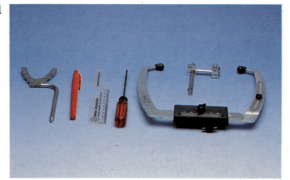

491 To mount the upper cast within the articulator the relationship of the occlusal surfaces of the upper teeth with the patient's nasion and external auditory meatus is recorded. To enable this to be done a bite fork (left), a face bow (right) and a means of joining them together (top right) are used. A handled spanner, a small measure and a marking pen are also required.

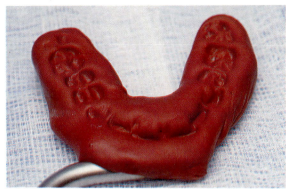

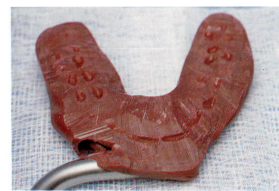

492 The first step is to cover the bite fork with softened composition and apply this to the occlusal surfaces of the upper teeth. The stem of the bite fork should be maintained in the centre line position.

493 When the upper model is mounted it is important to ensure that it is fully seated into the composition record or inaccuracies will occur. Any excess composition may mask whether this has been achieved and should therefore be trimmed away to leave only the tips of the cusps recorded. The accuracy of the composition can be improved by adding a trace of temporary cement to the cusp indentations and reseating the bitefork until the cement has set.

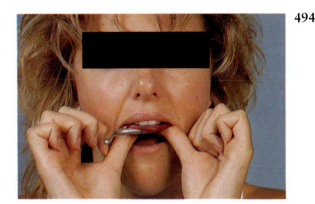

494 The patient's assistance is obtained to hold the re-seated bitefork firmly in place whilst the operator and chairside assistant attach the face bow to it.

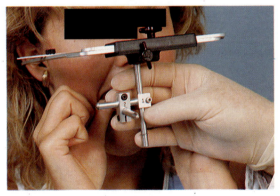

495 The ends of the face bow are placed into the orifices of the outer ear and the face bow is tilted so as to be a standard distance from the nasion. This is determined by marking the nasion with the coloured pen and measuring with the ruler.

   The fixing device is fitted to the underside of the face bow and also, by using the spanner, to the bite fork.

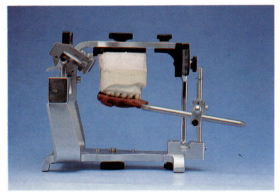

496 The upper cast, bite fork and fixing device are transferred to the articulator on to which the cast is mounted with plaster or dental stone. The upper arm of the articulator represents the cranium and the lower arch the mandible. Adjustments can be made to the hinge between the two to take account of patient variations in TMJ anatomy. These adjustments differ between designs of articulator and details are provided by the manufacturer.

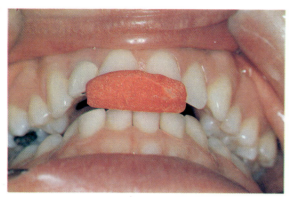

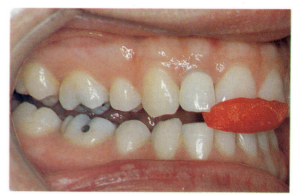

497, 498 It is now necessary to record the relationship between the lower and upper teeth so that the lower model can be mounted in the articulator to simulate accurately the patient's occlusion.

The relationship required is the retruded axis position i.e., when the mandibular condyles are both in their most posterior position with the upper and lower teeth just out of contact so that any influence from cuspal interference is avoided.

Getting the patient into the retruded axis position is the most crucial part of the technique and also the most difficult. The patient must be coaxed into relaxing and allowing the operator to position the mandible correctly, without resistance from the mastication muscles. This can be helped with a jig of self-curing acrylic adapted over the upper central incisors (**497**) and shaped with a palatal slope and stop which guides the mandible into the required position whilst holding the teeth slightly apart (**498**).

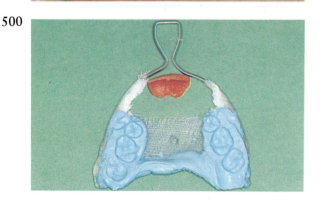

499 This position is recorded with impression paste. A horseshoe shaped wire frame is constructed which will lie in the buccal sulcus. Across its posterior half a piece of dental gauze is attached with sticky wax, taking care that this does not interfere with the anterior acrylic jig. The gauze is coated on both sides with just sufficient paste to record the upper and lower cusp tips when the patient closes into the retruded axis position, being guided there and maintained by the jig.

500

500 The jig and the occlusal record, when transferred to the mounted upper cast, will enable the lower cast to be mounted in its correct relationship.

If study casts are mounted in this way it will be possible to identify any occlusal interferences that are causing premature contacts or jaw deviations and adjust these before tooth preparation is undertaken.

Occlusal assessment of restorations

Interferences that did not exist before can, of course, be introduced by the new restoration; therefore careful assessment at the try-in stage is necessary to ensure that this has not occurred.

501 Very thin articulating paper is required for this assessment, such as GHM paper which can be obtained with marking ink on only one side thus keeping it as thin as possible. The marking ink is transferred from the paper to the tooth at any point of contact, provided the teeth are dry, and therefore marks such points very accurately.

Special tweezers are available for easier handling of this flimsy material which can be held in place by an assistant whilst the operator manipulates the relaxed jaw. This can be helpful in determining where premature contacts exist in centric occlusion.

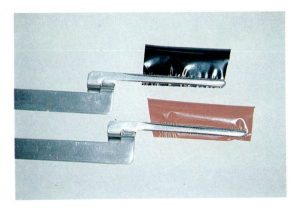

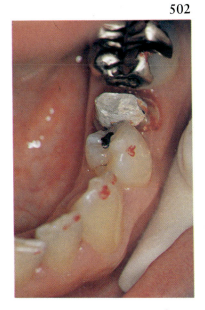

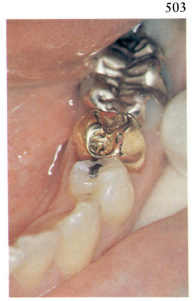

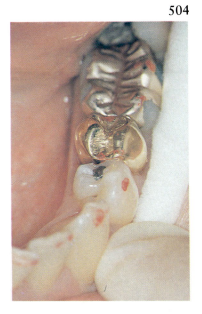

502 It is worthwhile, when trying-in any restoration, to establish what occlusal contacts exist between the patient's teeth when the restoration is out of the mouth. Centric protrusive and lateral contacts can be seen here marked in red.

503, 504 If these contacts are memorised and the marks removed, they should be repeatable with the restoration in place. If they are not (503) the only conclusion must be that the restoration is interfering with the proper contact of the teeth. The interference is marked red on the crown that is being tried on the second premolar and requires adjustment until the memorised contacts reappear (504).

505 A similar logic can be applied with shimstock, a sliver of exceedingly thin aluminium foil. Assessments are made of which teeth are able to grip the shimstock when the restoration is out of the mouth and when it is in place. If these do not correspond, the restoration must be high and will require adjustment before cementation.

A lifetime's supply of shimstock, 15 microns thick, can be obtained by passing a survival blanket through the office shredder.

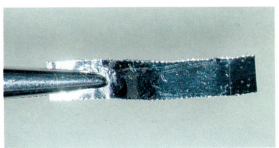

506

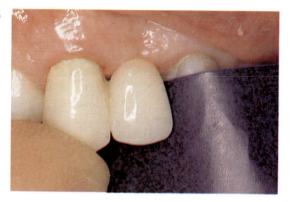

506, 507 At the try-in stage a crown or a bridge may not seat down because of tightness at the contact point area. A hit and miss approach to adjustment by the indiscriminate removal of porcelain or metal may well result in an open contact. It is, therefore, important to define the area of tightness precisely. This can be done using very thin articulating paper which is held interproximally whilst the crown or bridge is firmly seated into tight contact with the adjacent tooth (506). The area of tightness will be marked by the blue articulating paper (507) and can be reduced with accuracy.

507

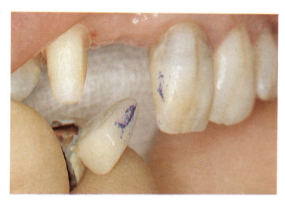

508

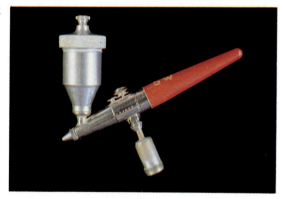

508 When a metal full veneer crown is being checked for tight contact points and occlusal interferences it is possible to reveal these with the aid of an airbrush. Demonstrated here is the Paasche airbrush (Paasche Air Brush Company, Chicago, USA.) which has been adapted to receive compressed air from the air line which normally drives the turbine handpiece. Activation of the button switch on the airbrush forces pumice powder from its reservoir in a fine jet through the nozzle.

509

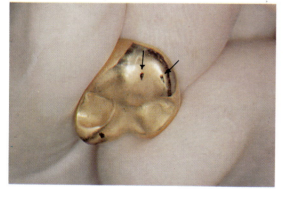

509 The stream of pumice particles is sufficient to put a bloom on the polished crown, without damaging its surface. Pressing the crown onto its preparation will reveal, by small burnished marks, any tight contacts that might be preventing it from seating. These can be eased very precisely. Once fully down the same procedure can be used to identify occlusal interferences (arrowed). This technique has the advantage of great accuracy because of the direct contact between crown and teeth, without the intervention of articulating paper. Some operators routinely ask their technicians to provide a bloomed surface rather than a polished one on their full veneer crowns.

16 Temporary coverage

If for any reason it is not possible to place a restoration immediately following tooth preparation, it is necessary to restore the tooth temporarily. The delay is usually due to the time required to construct an inlay, crown or bridge. Sometimes, however, it may be that time does not permit the insertion of an amalgam or composite filling which creates the need for a temporary dressing.

There are several reasons why temporary coverage of prepared teeth is required:

- Protection of the dentine from toxic irritation;
- Thermal insulation;
- Prevention of tooth movement;
- Prevention of food stagnation;
- Appearance.

In a retentive intra-coronal cavity, the simplest form of temporary dressing is provided by a stiffly mixed paste of zinc oxide powder and eugenol (ZOE) as used in stabilisation (see **63**). This will, however, take up to several hours to set fully and an accelerated proprietary version of ZOE cement may be preferred. If there is a danger that parts of such a dressing may break away, due to it not being adequately retained by what is left of the tooth, wisps of cotton wool may be incorporated in the mix to give added strength to the dressing. Gutta percha, which can be softened by heat, may be used as an alternative to ZOE. However, there is the risk of an inflammatory pulpal response when gutta percha is applied directly onto dentine. Its use should be restricted, therefore, to non-vital teeth or those where the dentine is already protected with a base.

Extra-coronal preparations may be protected with a variety of proprietary preformed temporary crowns or with ZOE supported by a copper ring. It is also possible to fabricate a custom made temporary crown or bridge either at the chairside or in the laboratory.

Anterior temporary crowns

These may be constructed in one of two ways; by use of a preformed crown shell refined, for a good fit, with an epimine resin or made entirely of epimine resin in an impression which acts as a mould to replicate the tooth's original shape.

Epimine resin is preferred to a self-polymerising acrylic resin because of its lower setting exotherm and its lower setting contraction. It is also less irritant to the gingivae and pulp.

A preformed temporary jacket crown

510–521 A polycarbonate crown is chosen, from the manufacturer's range, which matches as closely as possible the size and shape of the original tooth (**510**). The incisal tag, which carries the crown's type number, acts as a convenient handle for the crown during its adaptation to the preparation. This is twisted off and the incisal edge smoothed just prior to cementation.

It will be noted that the crown is too long by about 2–3mm and needs shortening by trimming

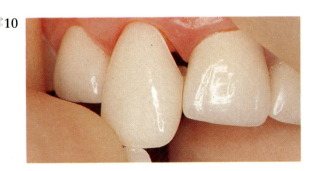

510

511

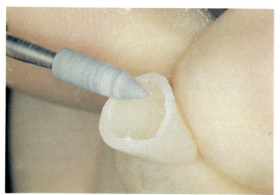

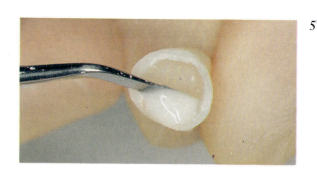

514

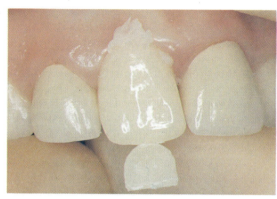

the cervical margin with crown scissors (**511**). This margin is smoothed and adjusted for a close cervical fit with a carborundum stone (**512**).

The crown form is filled with epimine resin (**513**), positioned accurately over the prepared tooth (**514**) and held steady until the resin has almost set. It is advisable to coat the preparation beforehand with a very thin film of lubricant to facilitate removal.

When the resin has set sufficiently to hold its shape, the crown is removed. A considerable excess will be noticed (**515**), but a good impression of the cervical margin of the preparation should be evident in the resin as confirmation of the accuracy of its fitting surface. The crown should then be placed in hot water to accelerate the completion of polymerisation whilst a thorough search is made for any excess epimine resin that might have been retained in the mouth. Being virtually transparent this is often difficult to detect.

515

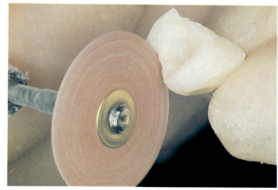

The cervical excess must be trimmed away to ensure a flush external fit that will not retain plaque and induce gingivitis. This can very readily be done with a sandpaper disc (**516**).

The crown is reseated and assessed for possible occlusal interference. This can be detected readily by a finger laid around the labial surfaces of the anterior teeth whilst the patient rubs the opposing

516

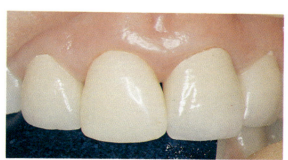

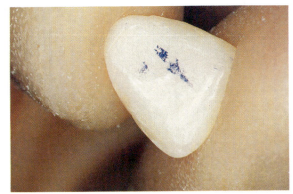

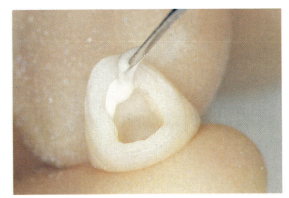
519

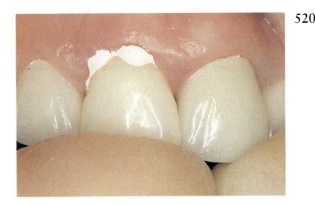
520

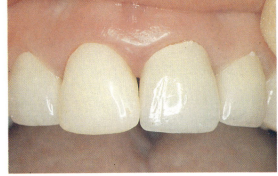

521

teeth over the palatal surface and incisal edge of the crown. Any independent movement of the crown indicates an interference, the commonest cause of its premature loss, and this must be removed. The area needing adjustment can be identified by articulating paper which is placed between upper and lower teeth (517) whilst the patient again rubs them together. The resulting marks of premature contact and protrusive interference (518) are removed and the procedure repeated until no new marks appear and normal contact is observed between adjacent upper and lower teeth.

A quick-setting temporary cementing medium is introduced into the crown (519) which is seated firmly into position in order to expel excess cement (520) and achieve the closest possible fit. If the cement is left undisturbed to set fully, it can be broken away cleanly to leave a smooth cervical finish (521). Dental floss should be introduced interproximally to remove the final traces of cement but care should be taken to withdraw this in a labial direction so as not to dislodge the crown.

Tailor made anterior crowns

A temporary crown exactly mimicking the original crown will obviate the need for time consuming adjustments. This can be achieved by taking an impression of the original tooth and its neighbours, either at the chairside or of a study model in the laboratory, before reducing it to a jacket preparation. If part of the crown has been lost due to caries or fracture it can be rebuilt with soft carding wax to provide its original shape for the impression.

When the preparation is complete, the appropriate part of the impression is filled with epimine resin and is seated firmly back in the mouth until the resin has set to a firm consistency. On removal of the temporary crown any excess is trimmed away after which it is fitted with a temporary cement.

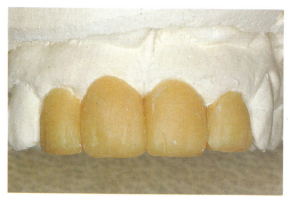

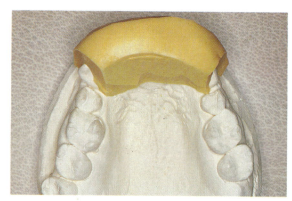

522 When several crowns are being provided, in this case for the four upper incisors which have become severely damaged by caries, the following technique is particularly useful. The desired shape for the jacket crowns is reproduced in wax by the laboratory.

523 An impression in silicone putty is taken of the waxed up crowns and adjacent teeth and is sent to the chairside.

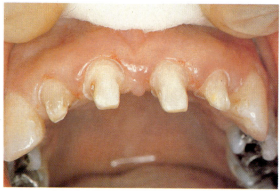

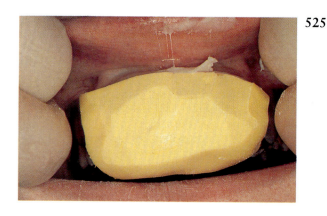

524 When the teeth have been prepared for jacket crowns and have been lightly lubricated, the incisor region of the impression is filled with epimine resin whilst taking care to avoid air inclusions.

525 The putty impression is seated fully over the teeth and preparations and is held steady until the resin is firm.

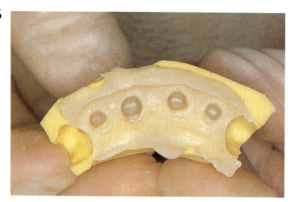

526 The resulting epimine 'impression' of the preparations is checked for completeness and full polymerisation aided by placing it in hot water.

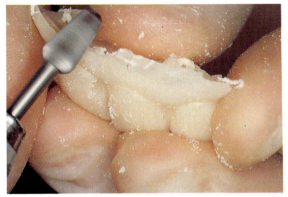

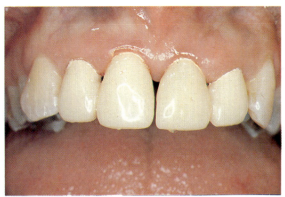

527 When the resin is fully hardened it is removed from the impression and the cervical excess removed.

528 The crowns are separated from each other with a fine disc or fretsaw and after smoothing interproximally they are inserted with a temporary cement.

A temporary post crown

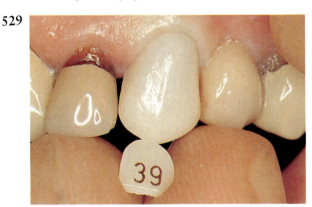

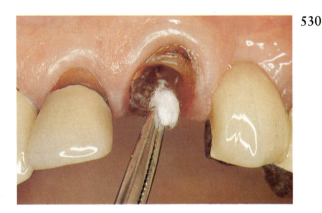

529 Temporary post crowns can also be constructed from preformed crowns or by using a putty impression of the original crown. In this example an appropriate polycarbonate crown has been chosen and tried in as before. It is trimmed to an accurate cervical fit.

530 If a temporary post, such as the Davis post, is to be used a small pinch of cotton wool is introduced to define the limit of the post hole and prevent the temporary cement uniting with the root filling cement.

531 If a full length and accurate fitting metal post is used, cotton wool will not be required. Some proprietary posts are manufactured with a 'nail' head but if the post is smooth the outer end of the post should be notched to aid retention between post and crown.

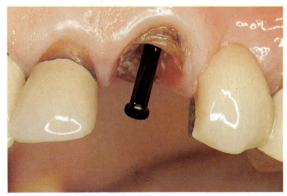

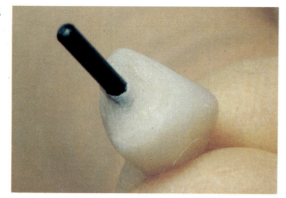

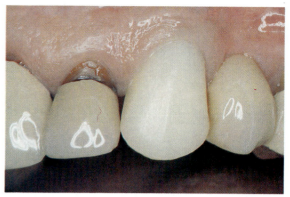

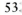

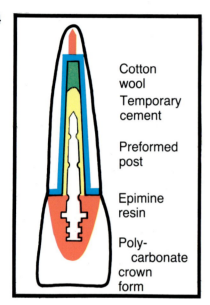

Cotton
wool

Temporary
cement

Preformed
post

Epimine
resin

Poly-
carbonate
crown
form

532 After filling the crown with resin it is seated over the temporary post and the resin allowed to set. Excess is trimmed leaving the post and crown ready for cementation.

533 Absence of gingival blanching and gentle probing confirms a flush fit with no cervical excess.

534 This line diagram illustrates the component parts of a temporary post crown made with a Davis preformed post.

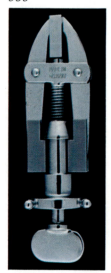   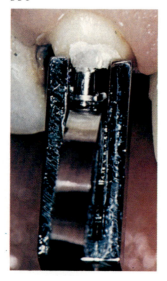

535, 536 A temporary post crown may be very well retained by the cement and to remove it by cervical leverage or extraction forceps may split the root or extract the tooth. The post can be more safely removed by drawing it out of the canal with an Eggler post remover (**535**).

In preparation for its removal the crown must be cut off the post which is then trimmed, if necessary, mesio-distally to allow the legs of the post remover to have access to the root face of the tooth. The jaws of the post remover are tightened onto the post by rotation of the capstan wheel. By turning the central screw the legs push against the root face (**536**) causing the jaws to draw out the post by breaking the cement seal.

Posterior temporary crowns

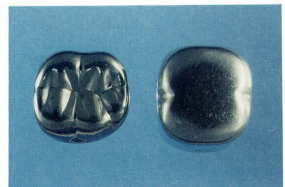

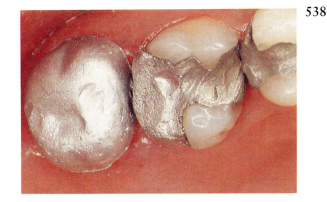

537–539 Full veneer crown preparations on posterior teeth can be covered temporarily with preformed aluminium crowns (537). These can be held in place with either a proprietary temporary cement or with ZOE. Aluminium crowns are supplied in two forms, one with full cuspal formation (left) and the other with a virtually flat occlusal surface (right). The anatomically shaped crowns are harder and stronger but the range of size and shape is limited. If it is not possible to find one which matches the tooth to be dressed, and which also has good contact points and an acceptable occlusal contour, it may be necessary to use the softer variety. One is chosen with a tight fitting circumference which is trimmed cervically to remove excess. Before cementation it is placed on the tooth so that the patient can mould the occlusal surface to an acceptable shape with their opposing teeth (538).

If care is not taken to achieve a good cervical fit, without sharp margins, gingival damage may be done which can leave the gums ulcerated and inflamed when the crown is removed (539). This will make it difficult to maintain a dry field when the permanent crown is being fitted.

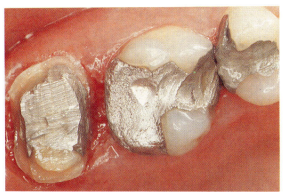

540 If the appearance of aluminium crowns is not acceptable , it may be preferable to use preformed polycarbonate crowns trimmed cervically, adjusted occlusally and cemented with a strong temporary cement. If a suitable preformed crown is not available it is possible to tailor make one in an epimine resin provided the operator anticipates the need and takes a silicone putty impression prior to tooth preparation.

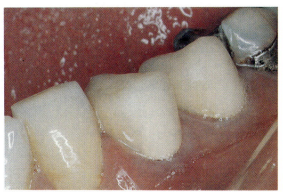

541

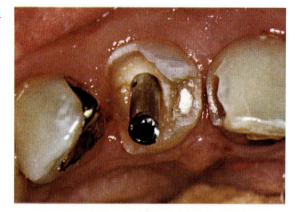

542

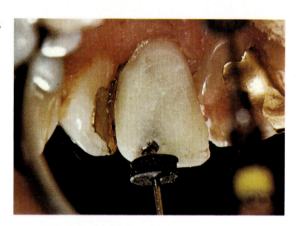

543

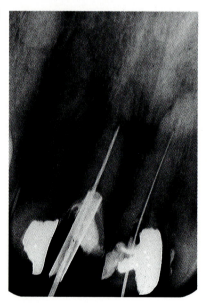

541–543 A temporary crown may be required for a badly broken down tooth which is undergoing root canal therapy. The crown can often be reformed temporarily with an acid-etched composite but if there is too little of the original crown left for its retention a post crown will be required. If the post used is a hollow one, root canal therapy can continue through it, obviating the need to remove and replace the crown at each visit. Orthodontic tubing will act as such a post. Its internal diameter should be greater than that of the biggest reamer likely to be used. An appropriate length of tubing is prepared and placed into a post hole that has been cut to a matching diameter (**541**).

A cellulose acetate crown form is trimmed to fit the root face and a hole cut in it to allow the orthodontic tubing to protrude. The outer end of the tube is blocked with cotton wool before the crown form, filled with epimine resin, is seated onto the tooth. When the resin has set the crown with its attached tubing is removed from the tooth and the cervical excess trimmed away. The protruding portion of the tube is reduced flush with the palatal surface and the completed temporary crown is cemented in place (**542**), taking care not to block the apical end of the tubing with cement.

Such a crown greatly assists the effective application of rubber dam thus preventing contamination. Furthermore, the creation of an incisal edge for the tooth provides a definite reference point from which to measure the working length for filing. A radiograph (**543**) demonstrates how instrumentation is possible with the crown in place.

17 Bridges

A bridge is defined in this book as a prosthesis which replaces missing teeth and is attached by means of cemented retainers to existing natural teeth. It is therefore not removable by the patient.

This distinguishes it from a small partial denture which is removable and which some people call a removable bridge.

Assessment

Spaces in the dental arch do not automatically qualify for filling with a prosthesis, there must be a good reason for this to be undertaken. One such indication might be a strong request by the patient for the space to be filled, either for aesthetic or functional purposes. Alternatively, the dentist may recommend action to prevent tilting or over-eruption of teeth (see **546, 547**).

If it is decided to provide a prosthesis a choice has to be made between a denture and a bridge. If the preference is for a bridge, several factors must be considered to determine if a bridge is a realistic possibility, and if so, what form its design should take (see Appendix 6).

Abutment teeth

A suitable number of abutment teeth are required to which the bridge can be attached. The number of abutments must be decided on an individual basis according to root morphology and anticipated occlusal load to which the bridge may be subjected.

The abutment teeth should have either vital and healthy pulps or sound and proven root fillings. If there is a choice it is preferable to use a tooth which has already been filled or crowned as an abutment rather than to severely reduce the crown of a completely sound tooth. It will, of course, be necessary to be satisfied that the restored tooth has a good prognosis. If an abutment tooth contains a large unpinned filling, it may be anticipated that the retention for this will be removed or considerably weakened during preparation for the bridge retainer. A pin retained filling should therefore be placed before the preparation is started.

Attrition and occlusion

Special note should be made of any signs of attrition as this will give an indication of where masticatory stresses are likely to be concentrated.

The occlusion should be assessed, preferably using study casts, for any cusps opposing the bridge which might cause occlusal interference or which might intrude into the space required by the pontic. These will need attention before a start is made on the bridge preparations.

Pontic area

The pontic area must be free of retained roots or buried teeth. If this point is overlooked, a future surgical operation may be impeded by the presence of the bridge, (see **624**).

147

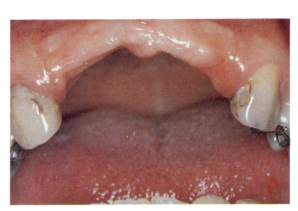

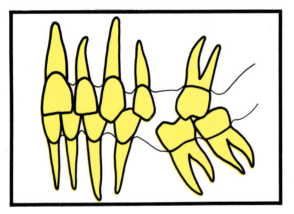

544, 545 For an anterior bridge, bone resorption in the pontic area must be minimal (**544**) to allow the pontic teeth to be gum-fitted in a pleasing manner. Where gross resorption has taken place (**545**) this will not be possible and an aesthetically acceptable result can only be obtained by reconstruction of the missing alveolus with pink acrylic in a partial denture or precision retained prosthesis.

Supporting structures

Bridges, being entirely tooth borne, rely for their support and retention on the abutment teeth via their roots and alveolar bone. Experience, rather than rules, must be relied upon for determining whether such support will be sufficient. The roots of the abutment teeth must be sufficiently long and substantial and the supporting tissues healthy enough to withstand the extra load that will be imposed upon them. A thorough clinical and radiographic assessment of these structures is therefore essential if an accurate prediction of the success of the bridge is to be made.

Choice of design

The various designs of bridge are classified in Appendix 6 and the choice is dependent on the availability of abutment teeth that satisfy the above criteria. If suitable abutments exist at each end of the pontic space, a fixed/fixed or fixed/moveable design would be appropriate. Indeed these are the commonest types of bridge in use. A cantilever design would have to be used if there was no suitable tooth at one end of the bridge span and a spring cantilever if the most suitable abutments were far away from the pontic area.

546, 547 Irreparable change may already have taken place in the supporting structures. Failure to maintain the space or spaces left after tooth extraction can lead to tooth movement unless this is prevented from occurring by existing intercuspal relationships. The teeth on either side of a gap may tilt into the space (**546**) or an opposing tooth may over-erupt (**547**). Either can result in occlusal interferences during functional excursions, and to periodontal deterioration.

Such consequences should and can be prevented if bridges or partial dentures are provided as soon as possible after tooth loss. Not every patient, however, will wish to accept a bridge following tooth extraction; it is neither economically realistic nor, in many cases, necessary. What is required is a means of assessing whether the dentition is stable after tooth loss or whether drifting is occurring. This can be achieved accurately with the aid of a succession of study models, at intervals of two or three months, from which measurements can be made. If small tooth movements have occurred it may be necessary to advise the patient of the need for a bridge. On the other hand if the teeth, through intercuspal contacts, are stable a bridge may only be necessary for reasons of appearance or masticatory function at the patient's request.

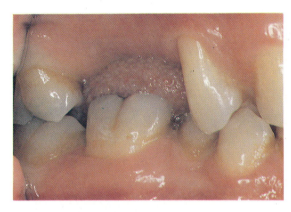

547

548 A useful alternative to a series of periapical radiographs for the assessment of a patient requiring bridges can be made with a rotational panoramic radiograph. This will give information about the bone support for the abutment teeth, the presence of roots or unerupted teeth in pontic areas and the direction of the long axes of the abutment teeth. It will also reveal periapical bone changes indicating the possibility of non-vital teeth. Other relevant information about the crowns of the abutment teeth, for example the extent of fillings, whether large amalgams are pinned, the presence of secondary caries, and the mesio-distal dimensions of the pulp chambers, is better provided by bitewing radiographs.

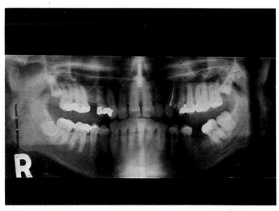

548

Fixed/fixed bridges

549 One of the commonest bridges is that which replaces a lower first molar. This tooth is often lost because of caries and the second molar is prone to tilt mesially. This tilting and possible over-eruption of the opposing molar can be prevented by means of a fixed/fixed bridge cemented to the teeth either side of the space. If aesthetically acceptable, this can be made most simply out of yellow gold with a full veneer crown as the retainer on the second molar and a three-quarter crown for the premolar. The pontic is a simple gold bar, fully functional but kept well clear of the mucosa to make the underside easy to clean.

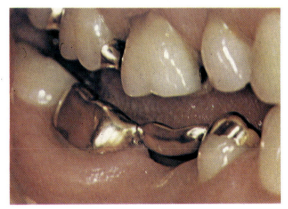

549

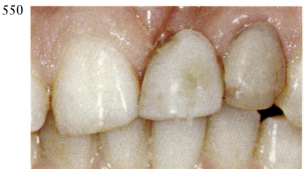

550

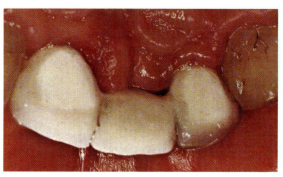

551

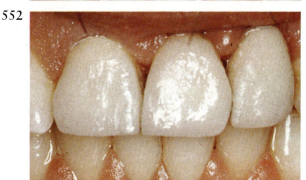

552

550–552 With the introduction of aluminous porcelain, great strength can now be obtained in the attractive looking all porcelain bridge. The discoloured acrylic crown on the lateral incisor and the partial denture replacing the upper left central incisor (550) are to be replaced with an aluminous porcelain bridge attached to the upper right central and the left lateral incisors, prepared for jacket crowns.

The palatal view (551) shows the distribution of the opaque aluminous cores which have been well masked in the labial view (552) by enamel and dentine type porcelain.

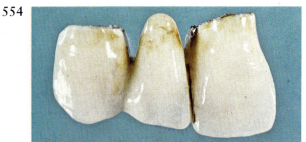

553

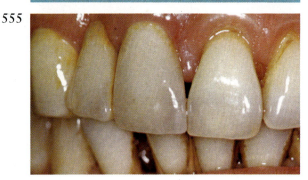

554

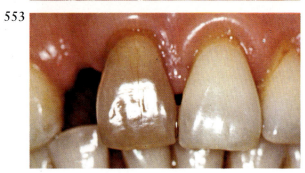

555

553–555 One of the problems with fixed/fixed anterior bridgework is the difficulty of disguising the fact that several teeth are joined together. In this example (553) the patient had a discoloured upper right central incisor and the adjacent lateral incisor is missing. Following the root filling of the central incisor, a cast post and core was fitted and the upper right canine reduced to a jacket crown preparation. A fixed/fixed all porcelain bridge (554) was made. The illusion of independent teeth was created by adding stain to the porcelain in the interdental areas. This allowed the tapered crown of the contralateral tooth to be copied without drawing attention to the connecting porcelain (555).

556 The ability to bond porcelain to metal makes it possible to construct much stronger anterior bridges, albeit sometimes at the expense of aesthetics. A layer of opaque porcelain is required to mask the underlying metal which, in its turn, requires covering with a considerable thickness of dentine and enamel porcelain to produce an acceptably natural appearance. This adds up to a total thickness of metal and porcelain of 1.5-2.0mm. As it may not always be possible safely to reduce the tooth to create this amount of space, the choice has to be made between making the restoration more prominent and bulky or trying to achieve an acceptable appearance with thinner porcelain.

Here the pontic replacing the first premolar is attached to full crowns on the canine and the second premolar. The resulting bridge looks rather dense and lifeless because of the problem of space.

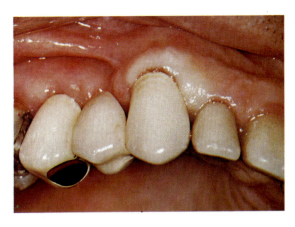

The gum around the canine is compressed and blanched and the cervical fullness will need reducing before the bridge is cemented.

557, 558 Replacement of a lower incisor with a bridge can be difficult if encroachment upon the tongue space is to be avoided. The lingual bulk can be kept to a minimum by coverage with metal alone (557). Only minimal reduction of lower incisors is advisable because of their small crown size and this reduction may not provide sufficient space for adequate labial porcelain coverage. However, any resulting labial fullness (558) is often better tolerated by the patient here than in the upper anterior region. With modern techniques it is probably more appropriate to consider the use of an adhesive bridge (see Chapter 18) if this will be acceptable to the patient's tongue.

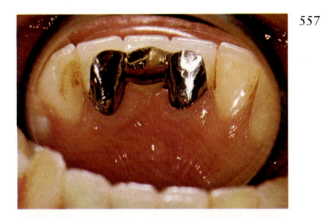

557

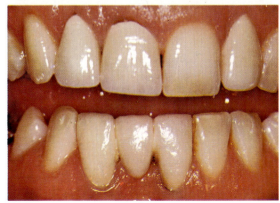

558

151

The problem of gingival recession

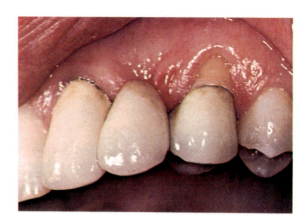

559 The bridge replacing the upper canine is attached to the lateral incisor and the first premolar by full coverage crowns. The pre-existing gingival recession, seen buccally on the premolar, would have presented two problems if an attempt had been made to finish the margin of the preparation subgingivally. Firstly the crown on the premolar would have looked excessively long. This could, however, have been disguised by shading the porcelain to make it match the cementum or even the gingivae (see **393**); but this solution would still leave the second problem, that of creating a shoulder of 1.5mm for metal and porcelain in this narrow root area, without exposing the pulp or seriously weakening the remaining tooth tissue.

The solution chosen was to finish the preparation at a supra-gingival level. Any slight darkening at the crown margin due to the underlying metal is usually well accepted by the patient as preferable to the risks of the alternative. If this is not acceptable the only solution would be to root fill the premolar and fit a post and core thereby allowing the margins of the bonded crown, suitably shaded, to be taken subgingivally.

Fixed/moveable bridges

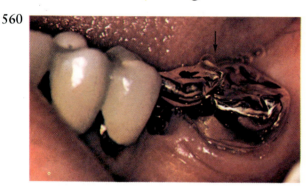

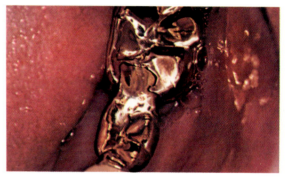

560, 561 This bridge replacing the first and second lower molars is retained by the first and second premolars and the third molar. The molar has tilted forward making it difficult to find a common path of withdrawal for the preparation of all three abutment teeth which would be necessary for a fixed/fixed design.

The bridge has therefore been designed to be in two parts. A full veneer gold crown has been made for the third molar with a line of insertion which matches its long axis. Within the mesial part of the crown, a slot has been created with a line of insertion that matches that of the two premolars. This slot accommodates a closely fitting dovetail projecting from the distal aspect of the pontic, which can be seen (**560**, arrowed) on this view showing the bridge partially inserted.

An occlusal view of the fully seated bridge (**561**) shows how the two parts of the bridge interlock. This design of bridge allows slight independent movement of the posterior retainer in only one direction and is thus almost as rigid as a fixed/fixed design.

Another application of this design is when two abutment teeth are of disparate sizes, typically a small premolar at one end and a large molar at the other. In these circumstances, some dentists prefer to introduce some stress breaking facility by means of a slot and dovetail at the minor or less retentive retainer, i.e. the premolar end of the pontic. This is claimed to reduce the risk of breaking the cement seal of the minor retainer during function.

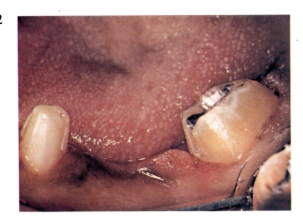

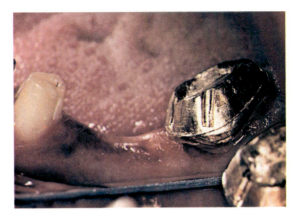

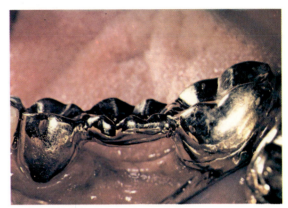

562–564 An alternative to the fixed/moveable solution to the tilted abutment problem is the 'telescopic' bridge which is particularly useful when the angle of tilt between the abutment teeth is severe (**562**). The molar retainer is made in two parts, the first (**563**) giving full coverage to the prepared molar. This is prepared with a line of insertion which suits its natural long axis whereas the outer contour of the gold coping is designed to simulate a full veneer crown preparation with a line of insertion compatible with that of the anterior abutment tooth. First, the gold cap is cemented to the molar, then the bridge itself is cemented in the usual way (**564**).

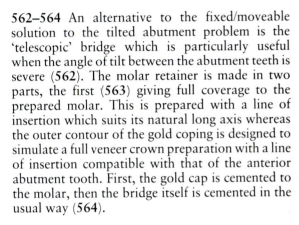

Simple cantilever bridges

565, 566 On occasions a suitable abutment tooth may not be available at both ends of a bridge span, or as in this case (**565**), it may be preferred not to involve the reasonably sound upper canine. A simple cantilever design can be adopted using the premolar and the previously crowned molar as abutment teeth. This example (**566**) shows how yellow gold and bonded gold can be combined by soldering the three units of the bridge together.

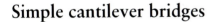

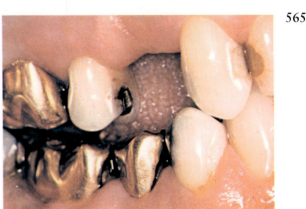

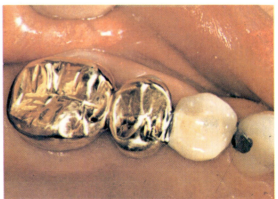

567

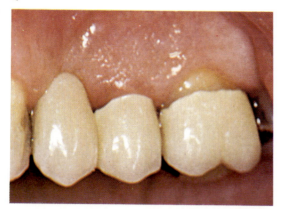

5•

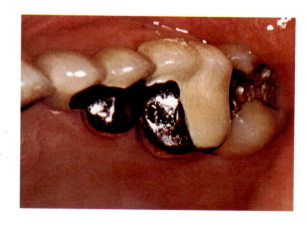

569

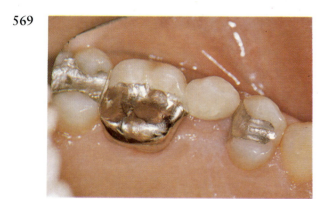

570

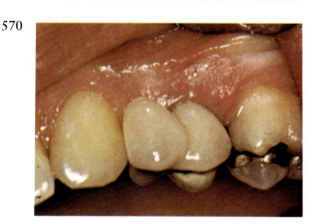

571

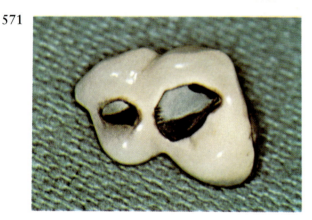

567, 568 An improvement to aesthetics can be achieved by making the whole bridge with a metal substructure, faced where appropriate with porcelain. Full coverage crowns on the second premolar and first molar carry a cantilever pontic to replace the first molar. The buccal margin of the molar retainer stops well short of the narrowing root (567). An occlusal view (568) shows that porcelain coverage has been omitted from areas of particularly heavy occlusal stress from opposing teeth. It also shows sites where attrition has made it imprudent to reduce the occlusal surface by the 2mm necessary to make room for porcelain as well as metal.

569 When the missing tooth is an upper second premolar, the first molar will often prove to be substantial enough to support a single abutment cantilever design of bridge, particularly if the pontic can be restricted to a simple buccal facade. This will reduce to a minimum any occlusal stress on the pontic.

570, 571 Here the space for the first premolar has partly closed and is not wide enough to admit a full sized tooth for a pontic. The situation can be disguised by placing a full width pontic slightly buccally to the arch and overlapping an apparently instanding second premolar. The effect of slight irregularity of the teeth (570) can be more pleasing to the eye than an overly small tooth fitted within the available space. The way that this has been achieved can be seen in 571. Because of the shortness of the pontic's span, it was not thought necessary to involve more than one abutment tooth.

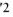

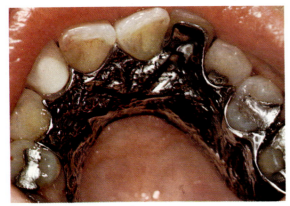

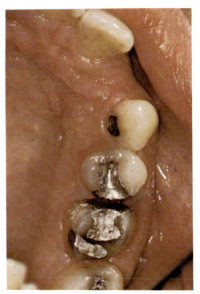

Spring cantilever bridges

572–575 This patient requested a bridge in place of the partial denture that carried the upper lateral incisor (**572**). After a full assessment of the possible abutment teeth and an analysis of the occlusion it was decided that the lateral incisor could be carried on the arm of a spring cantilever bridge attached to the first molar. This tooth was prepared for a full veneer crown (**573**). The fitted bridge compares favourably with the partial denture in its avoidance of gingival coverage (**574**) and gives a pleasing appearance (**575**).

The spring cantilever bridge is particularly useful in situations where diastemata would make it difficult to get an aesthetically acceptable result with a fixed/fixed bridge. Otherwise it has largely been superseded by the adhesive bridge.

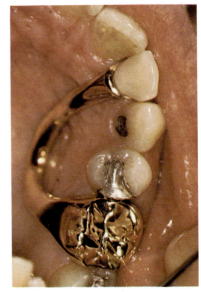

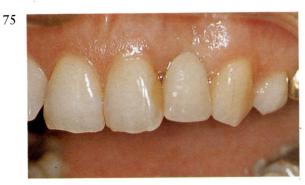

Compound and hybrid bridges

576, 577 Compound bridges combine two or more of the features of basic bridge design. I this example the absent lateral incisor and first premolar (**576**) are replaced with a five unit bridge composed of a simple cantilever pontic for the lateral and a fixed/fixed pontic for the first premolar.

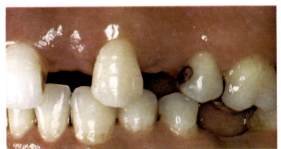

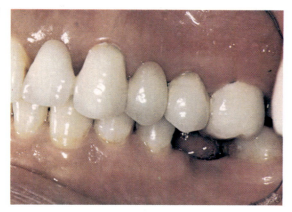

577

The canine, second premolar and first molar act as abutments (577).

578–582 A hybrid bridge combines elements of traditional bridge design with those of adhesive bridges (see Chapter 18). This patient had a badly discoloured upper right lateral incisor (578) and a missing upper right central replaced with an unsightly and bulky partial denture (579). These defects were remedied with a hybrid bridge which combined a Maryland restoration with a post crown (580).

After root filling, the lateral incisor was provided with a post and core (581). This was capped with a bonded crown containing a dovetail slot in its mesial surface. The pontic was attached mesially to the central incisor with a Maryland wing and was supported at the distal end by a dovetail which fitted into the bonded crown (582). In the event of the Maryland wing coming detached from the central it can be removed with the pontic and, after re-etching, be recemented.

578
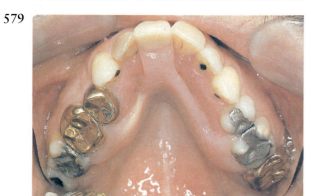

579

580
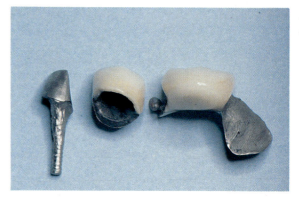

581
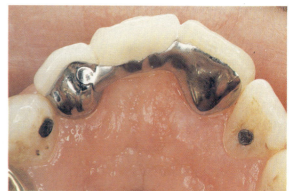

582

Temporary bridges

Once the final impression for a bridge has been taken, it is important to ensure that no tooth movement takes place while the bridge is being made. If any of the abutment teeth tilt, the parallelism achieved in the preparations will be disturbed and it will be difficult to insert the bridge. If adjacent teeth move towards the prepared abutment teeth, the resulting tightness in the contact areas will prevent the bridge from fully seating.

To prevent all these problems occurring and, of course, to cover exposed and sensitive dentine, it is necessary to fit an accurately constructed temporary bridge. This bridge must reproduce the original contours of the abutment teeth and also locks them together so that their relative positions, as recorded by the impression, are maintained.

The temporary bridge can be made at the chairside or in the laboratory, depending on the preference of the operator, the complexity of the bridge, available chairside time and the proximity of the dental laboratory.

583–586 This patient is to have the upper right canine replaced by a fixed/fixed bridge. The first step in the manufacture of a temporary bridge starts before any tooth preparation is undertaken. The missing canine is simulated in soft carding wax (**583**) and an impression of this is taken which also includes the unprepared surfaces of the abutment teeth. This impression, usually taken in a silicone putty, is set aside until the abutment teeth are prepared. The carding wax is removed and discarded.

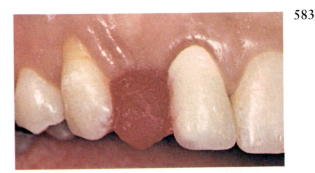
583

In this case the first premolar is prepared for a bonded crown retainer and the lateral incisor for a jacket crown retainer, using the existing core of the post crown (**584**).

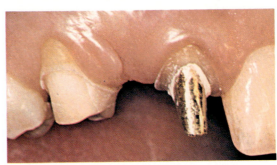
584

To make the temporary bridge the abutment and pontic aspects of the original putty impression are filled with a proprietary temporary bridge resin (**585**) taking considerable care to avoid any inclusions of air. The impression is re-seated firmly into the mouth so that the resin adapts itself closely to the previously lightly lubricated abutments. The outer surface of the resin takes up the shape of the original abutments and the waxed canine.

When the resin has set to a rubbery consistency the impression is removed, usually bringing the temporary bridge with it, and is transferred to hot water to accelerate the completion of polymerisation. The temporary bridge can now be taken safely from the impression without distortion and, after removal of all excess, is ready to be tried in for fit and lack of occlusal interference.

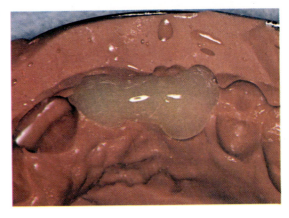
585

When satisfactory it is cemented in place with a temporary cement (586).

This technique has several advantages. By reproducing the exact contours that existed prior to treatment, occlusal equilibrium is maintained.

Furthermore the resulting temporary bridge will confirm, or otherwise, certain important aspects relating to the prepared teeth. The resin comprising the temporary bridge represents the amount of tooth tissue that was removed in preparing the abutment teeth. Enough should have been removed to create compatible withdrawal forms of the preparations and to give the laboratory sufficient scope to enable them to construct restorations that are no bulkier than the original teeth. If the temporary bridge cannot readily be removed from the abutment teeth this may well imply the existence of preparation undercuts or an incompatible path of withdrawal. If it is thin or even perforated occlusally or axially this will indicate insufficient reduction in these areas.

The temporary bridge needs to be made before the final impression is taken, so that any blemishes in tooth preparation can be revealed and adjusted.

586

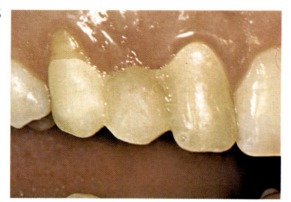

587

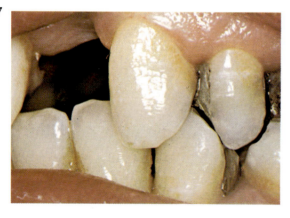

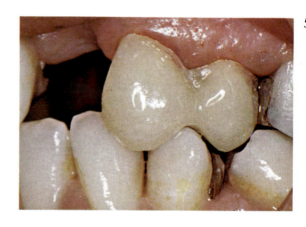

588

587, 588 If the space for the missing tooth is being maintained by a partial denture, or if the situation has been stable without space maintenance for some time, only the abutment teeth need to be included in the temporary coverage as in this case.

Laboratory made temporary bridge

The technician can make a temporary bridge in the laboratory, in heat or cold cured plastic or in cast metal such as silver. Such bridges will be stronger than those made at the chairside and may achieve a better finished result. It will be necessary for the dentist to provide study models on which the abutment teeth have been cut as closely as possible to the intended prepared shape.

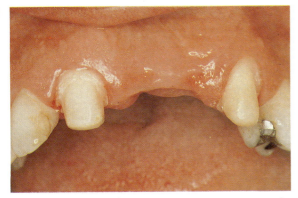

589

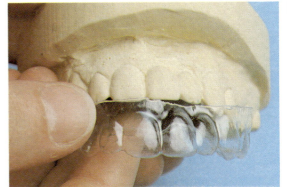

590

589–594 For an extensive bridge such as this which comprises all four incisors (**589**), it might be too time consuming to make the temporary bridge at the chairside and/or too difficult to get an acceptable appearance for the missing centrals with the carding wax technique.

A temporary bridge can be made in the laboratory from an upper impression taken of the almost completed abutment preparations. The technician waxes up the four incisors realistically (see **522**) and, after replicating the model, makes a mould for the temporary bridge from a plastic sheet by vacuum forming (**590**). A bridge resin is poured into the mould (**591**) which is applied to the original model after the wax has been removed and the preparations lightly lubricated (**592**). After removal from the model, considerable excess can be observed on the mucosal surface and cervical margins of the temporary bridge (**593**) which the technician can remove before sending it to the surgery. After refining the preparations and taking impressions for the working models the temporary bridge is fitted with a temporary cement (**594**).

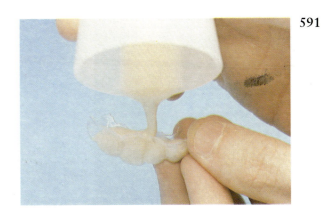

591

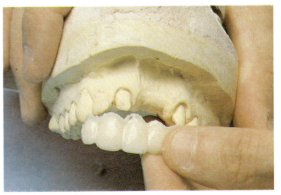

592

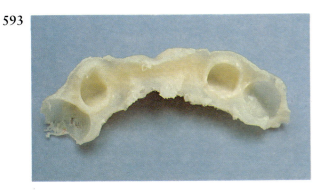

593

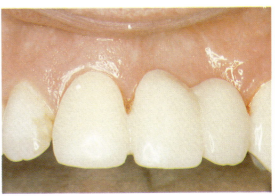

594

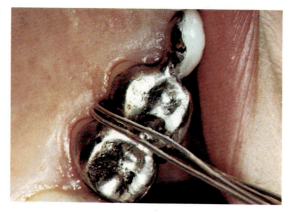

595

Bridge removal

595, 596 Plastic bridges can readily be prised or cut off the teeth but silver temporaries can be very retentive even with temporary cementation and cutting them can be time consuming. It is therefore worthwhile attempting to dislodge the bridge intact. This can often be done by feeding soft wire under the pontic or, as in this case (**595**) between the cantilever retainers, grasping the free ends of the wire with pliers and striking the pliers with a fist (**596**) to create a dislodging force in the line of withdrawal. This technique can also be used to remove an old bridge that is to be replaced but there is the risk of bringing cusps out with the bridge if force is exerted obliquely to the line of withdrawal.

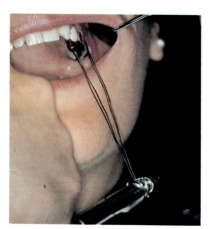

596

18 Adhesive bridges

It is possible, with modern materials and techniques, to attach metal castings to tooth enamel with composite resin. This has led to the introduction of new designs for bridges.

The composite cementing medium bonds to the enamel after it has been etched with phosphoric acid, and to the fitting surface of the metal when this has been suitably roughened to provide a mechanical lock. This rough surface is created in the laboratory in one of several ways, either before casting by treating the surface of the wax pattern or after casting by treating the metal.

The fitting surface of the wax pattern can be roughened by coating it with minute plastic beads which will burn out with the wax after investment for casting. Alternatively, crystals of common salt can be embedded in the fitting surface of the wax pattern which, when immersed in water prior to investment, dissolve leaving minute porosities in the wax. Both these methods provide good mechanical retention for the resin but the salt method, by virtue of creating porosities within the wax, enables the metal casting to be kept thinner than is possible when plastic beads are added to the wax surface.

More usually the cast metal is roughened either by air abrasion or electrolytic etching as in the Maryland design, whilst for a Rochette bridge, retention is obtained with a series of perforations.

It is advisable for the technician to coat the roughened fitting surfaces of an adhesive bridge with the thinnest possible layer of unfilled light-cured resin before the bridge leaves the laboratory. Besides saving chairside time, this will protect the fitting surface from becoming clogged with contaminants, particularly plaque or saliva, at the try-in stage.

It will be necessary to cement the bridge in place with a chemically or dual cured luting composite, since light will not penetrate the metal. It will, of course, reach the composite at the margins which enables it to activate the light cured component of the dual type composite. This can be very helpful, as the bridge can be 'tacked' in place quickly by light curing thereby keeping the bridge stationary whilst the bulk of the composite completes its chemical cure.

The big advantage of an adhesive bridge is that minimal reduction of abutment tooth tissue is required. Although this allows a very conservative approach to be adopted, by the same token the abutment tooth is made bulkier by the addition of metal to its surface. Careful assessment is required before treatment is started to ensure that this will not create any interferences with opposing teeth.

The retention of adhesive bridges though good, cannot match that of more traditional designs. This limits their use to single tooth spans in most cases and even then it is unwise to place one where the pontic will be subjected to excessive stress or to parafunctional habits.

597 To replace a missing lower incisor is notoriously difficult. A denture replacement is cumbersome, vulnerable to fracture, disadvantageous to the lingual gingivae and unwelcome to the patient.

A fixed/fixed bridge is usually preferred to a denture but the small crowns of the adjacent abutment teeth make reduction for full crown coverage hazardous.

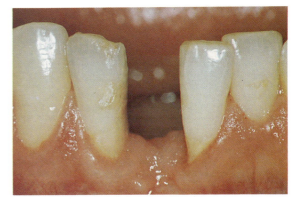

597

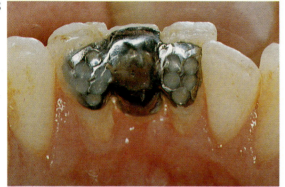

598 These problems were overcome with the advent of the Rochette design of adhesive bridges. Retention of composite to metal is achieved by perforating it with a series of small holes, made wider at their lingual ends, which enable the composite to 'rivet' the wings of the bridge to the abutment teeth. Because of the potential weakening effect of the perforations on the metal substructure the framework requires bulk and although in this case it is unlikely to interfere with the upper teeth, the patient may complain of encroachment into the tongue space.

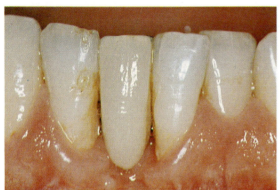

599 The pontic of porcelain bonded to the metal substructure gives a pleasingly realistic appearance if it can be gum-fitted. Care must be taken to ensure that its incisal margin is fractionally out of reach of the upper teeth. The patient should be instructed to floss daily using a floss threader and be warned to avoid biting heavily on the pontic.

600 In the Rochette design the 'rivets' of conventional composite also need considerable bulk for strength if they are not to fracture, and because of this it has been superseded in many instances by the Maryland design. Here the metal is not perforated and retention is obtained via its roughened fitting surface. This allows the metal wings to be kept much thinner which is of

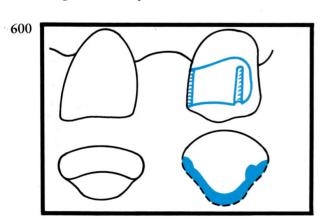

considerable benefit for a bridge replacing an upper incisor where clearance between abutment and opposing teeth may be minimal.

Space to accommodate the metal wing can be created by reduction of the palatal enamel (outlined in blue) however care must be taken not to expose the dentine. A simple cantilever design is often chosen to attach a small lateral incisor pontic to a substantial canine. This has the advantage of allowing the pontic to move with the abutment tooth thus avoiding the torque stresses that could be generated if it were to be fixed at both ends. Such stresses could break the bond to one or other of the abutment teeth and this, if unnoticed, will allow caries to develop between metal and tooth.

Tapered channels can be cut at both sides of the abutment tooth where the enamel is thick. These will add resistance form to the bridge and aid its location when it is cemented in place. The channels imply a vertical line of insertion and the preparation of the palatal enamel and any channels must be consistent with this direction in order to avoid undercuts.

601–603 A single abutment design is not usually recommended for the replacement of a central incisor because of the risk of rotation of an incisor by leverage on the cantilevered pontic. The area of enamel reduction has been marked on the working model (**601**), and the cingulum area on each tooth has been reduced to a flat table. This will aid the location of the bridge during cementation and give resistance to dislodgement from shearing stresses.

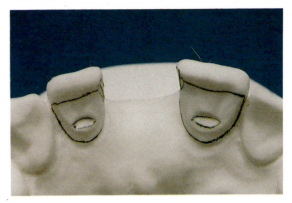

It will be seen from the palatal view (**602**) of the fitted bridge that the cingulum reduction has created space for stops to be introduced for the occlusion of the lower teeth. These will ensure that occlusal force is directed in the long axis of each abutment tooth thus reducing the tendency to cause proclination.

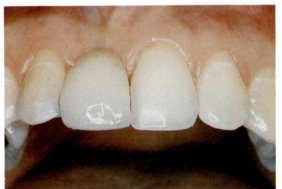

The labial view (**603**) demonstrates that if the palatal metal-work of the retaining wings is confined to the thicker parts of the teeth, it does not show through the porcelain incisal tips (compare with **630**).

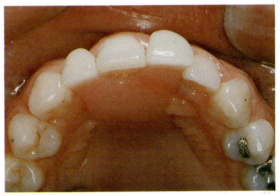

604–608 This patient with a bulky acrylic denture replacing the upper right lateral and left central incisors (**604**) requested its replacement by a bridge.

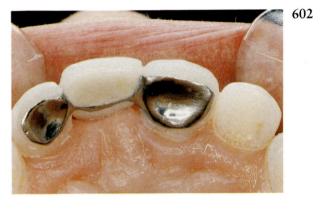

605

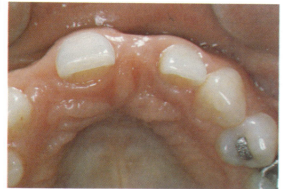

The surrounding teeth were perfectly sound (605) and their reduction for full crown coverage was not justified. Occlusal clearance existed for the placement of an adhesive bridge and as the two teeth to be replaced were separate single tooth spans, a 5 unit bridge (606) was considered appropriate. Note the incisal hooks of metal on the outer wings. These ensure the accurate positioning of the bridge and are removed after cementation (607, 608). The favourable occlusal relationship between the upper and lower incisors has facilitated the success of this bridge.

606

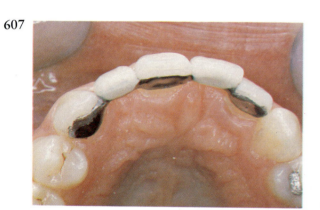

609 Adhesive bridges are proving both successful and conservative restorations for replacing single posterior teeth. Here the occlusal stresses to which they are subjected are much greater than for anterior bridges and so this must be taken into account when designing the bridge.

The wings of the bridge must embrace as much of each abutment tooth as possible for maximum retention. This 'wrap-around' effect is achieved by removing enamel from as much as half the circumference of each crown as aesthetics and the adjacent teeth will allow (top, cross-hatched blue).

An occlusal rest seat is cut in each abutment in the pontic region (top and bottom, solid blue) and a retentive location channel at the remote end of each wing. The lower diagram shows the way that the lingual bulbosity must be reduced to eliminate undercuts.

607

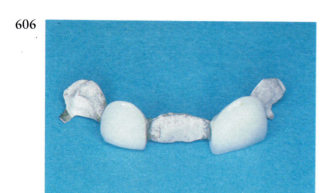

608

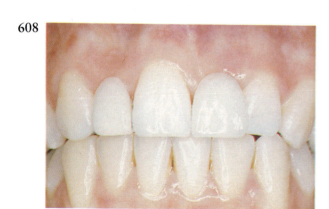

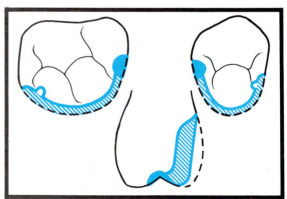

609

610, 611 The enamel reduction has been outlined on this working model in pencil. Retention channels may be placed additionally or alternatively below the rest seats (**610**). With good 'wrap-around' and retentive channels a posterior bridge should have sufficient retention to stay in place (**611**) during the try-in whilst the occlusion is checked for all excursions of the mandible.

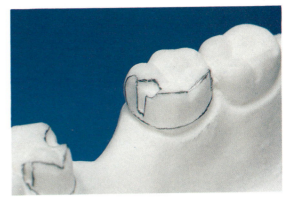

610

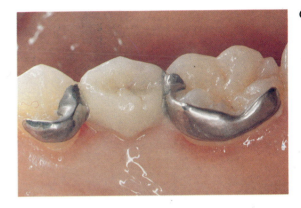

611

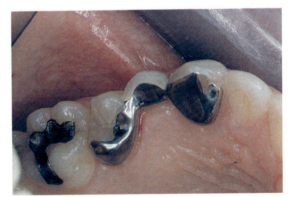

612

612 For replacement of an upper first premolar an adhesive bridge design may incorporate both anterior and posterior bridge features as seen in this example; the bridge is attached to the canine abutment with a cingulum wing and to the second premolar with a 'wrap-around' wing and cingulum rest.

19 Some errors and problems in bridgework

613 Special attention must be paid to the contour and design of the fitting surfaces of pontics in order to allow thorough cleaning with dental floss or other plaque removing agents. Wherever possible these surfaces should be convex, because strongly concave surfaces are not very accessible. When the upper anterior bridge was removed from this patient the mucosa was found to be grossly inflamed. This proved to be the result of over-extended and poorly contoured pontics.

Whilst it is not always possible to achieve convexity, any concavity should be kept to a minimum so that it can be reached by a thickened floss, such as Superfloss (Oral-B, Redwood City, C.A. 94065 USA).

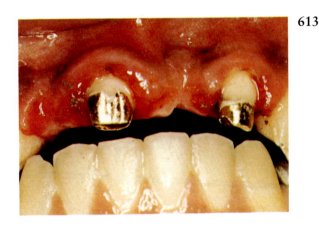

613

614, 615 Gingival problems can also arise if the interproximal contours of retainers do not allow sufficient space to accommodate the gingival papillae. The porcelain of these two retainers (**614**) is united from incisal to gingival margins thus crowding out the papillae. This should be avoided by presenting the technician with a full prescription for the bridge which includes information about gingival levels and contours. The bridge has been improved by re-contouring the porcelain interproximally (**615**) but in doing so the glaze will have been removed. It is important that the resulting plaque retentive surface is re-glazed or highly polished with polishing discs and rubber wheels and points.

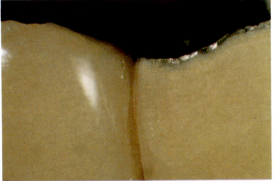

614

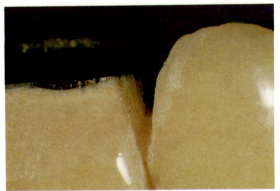

615

616

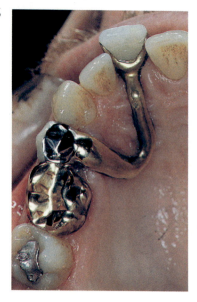

616 If a bridge is not correctly designed or strongly constructed there is the risk that the pontic may be displaced. This example reveals a spring cantilever bridge whose arm supports the central incisor pontic and is attached to the second premolar and first molar. The central pontic has been displaced upwards and labially allowing the adjacent teeth to close towards each other. The reason for this displacement can be seen to be heavy occlusion from the lower incisors onto the bar of the spring cantilever arm. A facet of wear has weakened the arm and allowed it to distort.

617

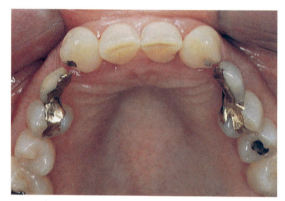

617 This patient had missing upper lateral incisors which resulted in the canines erupting into contact with the centrals. The spaces between canines and first premolars have been filled by simple cantilever pontics attached to mesio-occlusal inlays in the first premolars. The design for both bridges incorporated an occlusal rest which did not lock firmly into the canine. As a consequence both canines have moved labially. The bridges were made of medium yellow gold which was not strong enough to withstand occlusal stresses. The pontic on the right has been bent palatally and the occlusal rest on the left has been broken off. Inlays as retainers for bridges have been shown to be inadequate (Roberts, 1970), and any gold other than hard gold is likely to distort under the extra loads imposed by a bridge.

618

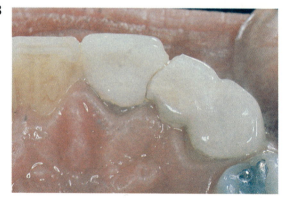

618 Bridges made entirely of porcelain are vulnerable to fracture. With a thorough initial assessment it may have been possible to predict the outcome, indicating to the operator the need for a design using a stronger material. Where doubt exists it is probably wise to select porcelain bonded to metal for such a bridge.

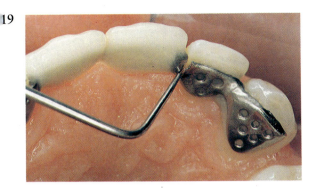

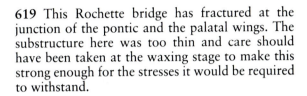

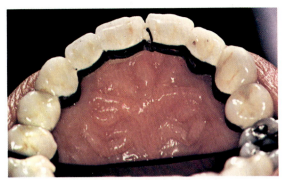

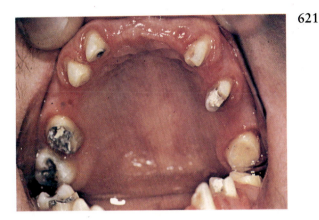

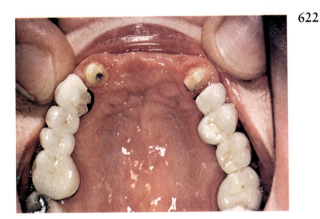

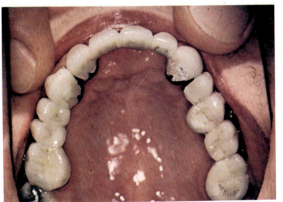

619 This Rochette bridge has fractured at the junction of the pontic and the palatal wings. The substructure here was too thin and care should have been taken at the waxing stage to make this strong enough for the stresses it would be required to withstand.

620–623 Even conventional bridges with metal substructures can fracture (**620**). This fracture may have been due to a flaw in the casting or due to the unyielding nature of a 10-unit bridge made in one piece. All ten units will have to removed unless the distribution of abutments allows the broken portion to be sectioned and remade independently of the other parts.

It would have been sensible to make such an extensive bridge in separate parts in the first place. Here six abutments are available to support pontics in four areas (**621**). The abutments are placed so that it has been possible to replace the posterior teeth with a fixed/fixed bridge on the right and a compound fixed/fixed and simple cantilever bridge on the left (**622**). The anterior fixed/fixed bridge completes the restoration of the upper arch (**623**). Such an approach allows some independent movement between the three components which will reduce the likelihood of fatigue fracture. Should any problem occur making replacement necessary, it will be confined to one section out of the three. If it is thought necessary to interlock all three sections, an impression can be taken over them at try-in stage. They can then be returned to the laboratory for the incorporation of precision attachments.

624

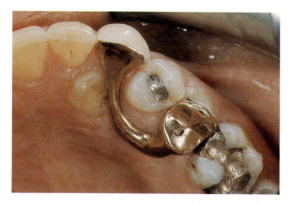

624 This is a case of bad planning. A bridge has been made to fill the gap between the lateral incisor and first premolar without using radiographs to determine the fate of the canine. At the time it was unerupted and its removal now is seriously impeded by the presence of the bridge.

625

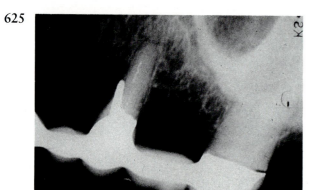

625 Although this bridge has been compromised by the perforation of the root of the second premolar when preparing its canal to receive a post and core, the patient's complaint was typical of pulpits centred on the upper molar. Radiographic evidence indicates that the full crown retainer has become detached from the abutment tooth with loss of cement allowing dentine irritation to occur.

626

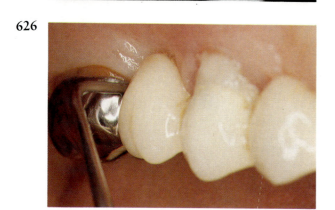

626, 627 One does not always get such clear cut help from a radiograph and it may be difficult to determine whether a retainer has become loose or not. Sometimes movement of the retainer relative to its abutment can be detected if an instrument which is inserted under the pontic (**626**) is able pull the retainer in an occlusal direction. Alternatively finger pressure, applied occlusally to the suspect retainer, may cause bubbles of air and saliva to escape from around the margin of the crown (**627**).

627

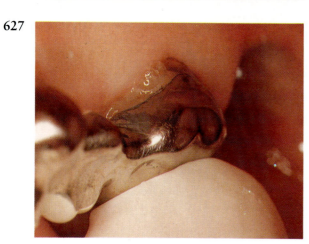

628, 629 The bridge replacing the upper first molar was removed from this mouth because the distal retainer had been found to be detached from its abutment. Rampant caries of the second molar can be seen to be the consequence of this detachment (**628**), the bridge, unfortunately, having been retained by the premolar which was quite sound.

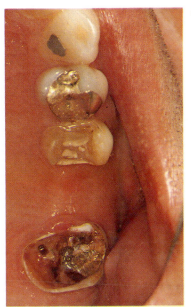

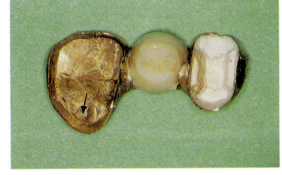

On examination of the fitting surfaces of the bridge retainers, that for the molar was seen to be devoid of cement (**629**). Closer inspection revealed an occlusal perforation of the gold (arrowed) and this had allowed the cement to leach out. This emphasises the need for hard gold to be used in bridgework with sufficient occlusal reduction being made during tooth preparation to allow an adequate thickness of gold coverage. By contrast, the cement in the premolar retainer was intact.

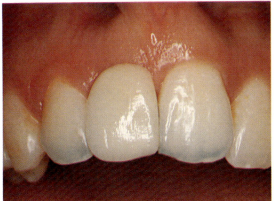

630 Although adhesive bridges can give excellent aesthetic results care must always be taken to avoid the metal wings from showing through the incisal enamel as they have done in this example on the right lateral and left incisor. This can be assessed before deciding on the design of the retentive wings, by holding a metal instrument behind the incisal tips of the abutment teeth.

20 Monitoring and maintenance

Although fillings and restorations are described in dental terminology as temporary or permanent, it is a fact that 'permanent' fillings are incorrectly named. Very few restorations last a patient's lifetime. Studies have shown that the average life of an amalgam restoration, for instance, is 8–10 years (Qvist *et al.*, 1986). This implies that a filling placed in the tooth of a patient aged 15 is likely to be replaced at least five times by the age of 65.

Even with extreme care it is difficult to replace a filling without increasing the size of the original cavity and this, together with any enlargement required to deal with recurrent caries, can readily weaken the remaining tooth tissue so that cuspal or even whole tooth fractures occur.

It is, therefore, important for the dentist to ensure that a very pressing reason exists for the replacement of a restoration so that the number of such occasions is kept as low as possible. Furthermore, if interference is justified this should be kept to the absolute minimum. It used to be the practice to recommend the total replacement of any filling that did not match the textbook ideal. It is now an accepted maxim that if doubt exists, one should wait and see, and if there is no doubt, repair should be considered in preference to total replacement.

All restorations should therefore be monitored at intervals appropriate for a particular patient. These intervals may vary between 6 months and 2 years dependent on factors that influence the initiation and rate of dental caries. An interval of 6 months may be chosen for a young patient in the caries prone age group or a patient whose diet or plaque control is suspect. The interval for older patients, in good periodontal health, who have shown little or no primary or recurrent caries at 6 monthly recalls, may be increased to 1 or even 2 years. Patients who are periodontally suspect, or who wear a removable prosthesis should be monitored more frequently.

Bitewing radiographs should be taken, dated and retained at each monitoring session and a careful record made of all sites where caries is suspected. Only in this way can a comparison be made at the next check-up and a valid opinion formed as to whether the caries is progressing, arrested or even remineralised

Amalgam restorations

Amalgam restorations are prone to show defective margins after a year or two of service. This 'ditching', as it is called, can be the result of loss of marginal enamel, fracture of the amalgam or a combination of both. The risk can be reduced if care is taken at cavity preparation to prepare butt-joint margins thus avoiding unsupported enamel. The use of the stronger high-copper amalgam alloys will reduce the likelihood of creep, a potent factor in fractured amalgam margins. In addition good moisture control will prevent delayed expansion of the amalgam which can also encourage marginal fracture.

Nevertheless, ditching can occur but this in itself is not sufficient reason to replace the filling. Interference is only justified if there are symptoms or if retention of plaque has caused caries to develop and then only if preventive measures fail to arrest the lesion.

If caries does progress, it is necessary to establish whether this is universally affecting all margins or extensively involving the dentine before total replacement is justified. If caries is confined to a section of the filling's perimeter a repair can be undertaken with amalgam, glass ionomer or cermet material. The carious tissue should be removed with the smallest fissure bur available and as far as possible at the expense of the existing filling. If amalgam is to be used for the repair, slight undercut is required in the repair cavity. This is not necessary in the case of glass ionomer or cermet as these will both adhere to tooth tissue and to freshly cut amalgam (Aboush and Jenkins, 1989).

Involvement of dentine by recurrent caries may be suspected if colour changes appear through the surrounding enamel, although this can be confused with colour changes produced by the amalgam itself or its corrosion products. A bitewing radiograph may resolve this dilemma but it must be noted that caries can be masked by the radio-opaque amalgam. If doubt exists, the tooth can be put on probation until the next recall. If there are multiple suspect amalgams it may be justifiable to remove one to confirm whether caries is present or not. This can help in deciding whether to replace other fillings.

Caries may not, however, be the problem. The amalgam or a cusp may have fractured. Again, careful consideration should be given to the possibility of repair rather than total replacement (Cowan, 1983).

The cusps of premolars with wide MOD amalgam restorations are particularly vulnerable to fracture. It is not realistic to restore with a full veneer crown every tooth that has a fractured cusp. Satisfactory repair can be achieved with glass ionomer or a glass ionomer base faced with composite. If appearance is not a limiting factor, amalgam can be used and retention provided by the combination of a pin and a small dovetail interlocked into the existing amalgam.

A Class II amalgam with a fractured keyway may sometimes be repaired by removal of amalgam from the interproximal box alone and then interlocking into the existing amalgam. However, the cause of the original fracture must be diagnosed. This will often be because of shallowness in the original cavity in which case total replacement, after suitable cavity modification, will be necessary.

A complaint of food packing is often due to an open contact between a Class II amalgam restoration and the adjacent tooth. Wherever possible this should be dealt with by adding amalgam interproximally, by a similar technique to that used for a fractured amalgam, thus avoiding unnecessary loss of sound tooth tissue.

Cervical amalgam excess, usually only revealed on bitewing radiographs, is often impossible to remove effectively because of difficulties of access. Even if removal were achieved the remaining amalgam, due to its poor condensation, would be porous and difficult to keep free of plaque. In this case removal of the filling, at least from the box, would be justified.

Composite restorations

Composites are used predominantly in sites where appearance is a factor. Any discoloration is thus likely to bring forth a complaint from the patient. Many of the early composites changed colour in time but modern materials have largely overcome this problem and are colour-fast. Discolouration can occur, however, due to superficial staining where the composite has lost its initial glaze or polish and around the margins where edges have been left or where acid-etching has been inadequate.

Such defects rarely warrant total replacement of the composite. Discolouration due to surface roughness can be remedied by re-polishing with discs. This will restore the appearance and leave the surface less likely to discolour in the future.

Marginal discolouration, whether due to staining or recurrent caries cannot always be removed without leaving the restoration deficient and prone to plaque retention. However, as new composite will adhere to old it will usually only be necessary to skim the outer layer of composite and reface it, without the need for total replacement. It is wise to freshen up the adjacent enamel, re-etch and apply unfilled resin, before adding the new composite. This will ensure good marginal seal and reduce the risk of further discolouration.

Posterior composite used in wide cavities in premolars and molars can be susceptible to wear, although modern materials have greatly reduced this risk. If wear does occur it can be followed by over-eruption leading to occlusion problems and difficulties for future restoration of the teeth involved. This needs careful monitoring and, where necessary, treatment before irreversible changes take place.

References

Aboush, Y.E.Y. and Jenkins, C.B.G. (1989). The bonding of glass ionomers to dental amalgam. *Brit. Dent. J.*, **166**, 255–257.

Ainamo, J. and Bay, I. (1975). Problems and proposals for recording gingivitis and plaque. *Int. Dent. J.*, **25**, 229–235.

Ainamo, J., Barmes, D., Beagrie, G., Cutress, T., Martin, J., and Sardo-Infirri, J. (1982). Development of the World Health Organisation (WHO) Community Periodontal Index of Treatment Needs (CPITN). *Int. Dent. J.*, **32**, 281–291.

Baker, D.L. and Curson, I. (1974). A high speed method for finishing cavity margins. *Brit. Dent. J.*, **137**, 391–396.

Berman, D.S. and Slack, G.L. (1973). Caries progression and activity in approximal tooth surfaces. *Brit. Dent. J.*, **134**, 51–57.

Boyde, A., Knight, P.J. and Jones, S.J. (1972). Further scanning electron microscope studies of the preparation of Class II cavities. *Brit. Dent. J.*, **132**, 447–457.

Britton, A.S. (1976). Total coronal pulpotomy of the vital permanent molar. *Proc. Brit. Paedodontic Soc.*, **6**, 15–18.

Cameron, C.E. (1964). Cracked tooth syndrome. *J. Am. Dent. Ass.*, **68**, 405–411.

Cameron, C.E. (1976). The cracked tooth syndrome: additional findings. *J. Am. Dent. Ass.*, **93**, 971–975.

Cowan, R.D. (1983). Amalgam repair - A clinical technique. *J. Prosth. Dent.*, **49**, 49–51.

Elderton, R.J. (Editor) (1975). Research on cavity design for amalgam restorations. *Proc. Int. Symp. on Amalgam and Tooth-Coloured Restorative Materials*, p. 241, University of Nijmegen.

Elderton, R.J. (Editor) (1990). Principles in the management and treatment of dental caries. *The Dentition and Dental Care*, Chapter 13, p. 244, Butterworth Heinemann, Oxford.

Fisher, F.J. (1972). The effect of a calcium hydroxide/water paste on micro-organisms in carious dentine. *Brit. Dent. J.*, **133**, 19–21.

Gwinnett, A.J. (1971). A comparison of proximal carious lesions as seen by clinical radiography, contact microradiography and light microscopy. *J. Am. Dent. Ass.*, **83**, 1078–1080.

Gwinnett, A.J. and Buonocore, M.G. (1965). Adhesives and caries prevention: a preliminary report. *Brit. Dent. J.*, **119**, 77–80.

Masterton, J.B. (1966). The healing of wounds of the dental pulp of man. A clinical and histological study. *Brit. Dent. J.*, **120**, 213–224.

McLean, J.W. and Gasser, O. (1985). Glass-Cermet cements. *Quint. Int.*, **16**, 333–343.

McLean, J.W. and Sced, I.R. (1976). The bonded alumina crown: 1. The bonding of platinum to aluminous dental porcelain using tin oxide coatings. *Aust. Dent. J.*, **21**, 119–127.

Messing, J.J. and Stock, C.J.R. (1988). *A Colour Atlas of Endodontics*, Wolfe Publishing Ltd., London.

Mooser, M. (1970). A standardised pin anchorage. *Quint. Int.*, **1**, No.12. p.23

Newsome, P.R.H. (1988). An alternative to pins and posts in the restoration of rootfilled molar teeth. *Rest. Dent.*, **4**, 38–42.

O'Leary, T.J., Drake, R.B. and Naylor, J.E. (1972). The plaque control record. *J. Perio.*, **43**, 38–40.

Podshadley, A.G. and Haley, J.V. (1968). A method for evaluating oral hygiene performance. *Pub. Health Rep.*, **83**, 259.

Qvist, V., Thylstrup, A. and Mjor, I.A. (1986). Restorative treatment pattern and longevity of amalgam restorations in Denmark. *Acta Odontol. Scand.*, **44**, 343–349.

Roberts, D.H. (1970). The failure of retainers in bridge protheses: An analysis of 2000 retainers. *Brit. Dent. J.*, **128**, 117–124.

Shortall, A.C., Bayliss, R.L., Bayliss, M.A. and Grundy, J.R. (1989). Marginal seal comparisons between resin bonded Class II porcelain inlays, posterior composite restorations and direct composite resin inlays. *Int. J. Prosth.*, **2**, 217–223.

Taggert, S.E. and Pearson, G.J. (1988). The effect of etching time on glass ionomer cement. *Rest. Dent.*, **4**, 43–47.

Tronstad, L. and Leidal, T.I. (1974). Scanning electron microscopy of cavity margins finished with chisels or rotating instruments at slow speeds. *J. Dent. Res.*, **53**, 1167–1174. ibid (1975) - finished with ultraspeed instruments. *J. Dent. Res.*, **54**, 152–159.

Wilson, C.A. and Tay, W.M. (1977). Alum solution as an adjunct to gingival retraction. A clinical evaluation. *Brit. Dent. J.*, **142**, 155–158.

Recommended textbooks

Baum, L., Phillips, R.W., and Lund, M.R. (1985). *Textbook of Operative Dentistry*, 2nd Edn., W.B. Saunders Co., Philadelphia.

Cohen, S. and Burns, R.C. (1991). *Pathways of the Pulp*, 5th Edn., Mosby–Year Book, Inc., Missouri.

Deubert, L.W. and Jenkins, C.B.G. (1982). *Tooth-coloured Filling Materials in Clinical Practice. Dental Practitioner Handbook*, 16, 2nd Edn., John Wright & Sons Ltd., Bristol.

Eccles, J.D. and Green, R.M. (1983). *The Conservation of Teeth*, 2nd Edn., Blackwell Scientific Publications, Oxford.

Elderton, R.J. (Editor) (1990). *Clinical Dentistry in Health and Disease*. Vol. 3, The dentition and dental care, Heinemann Medical Books, Oxford.

Harty, F.J. (1990). *Endodontics in Clinical Practice. Dental Practitioner Handbook*, 24, 3rd Edn., John Wright & Sons Ltd., Bristol.

Jordan, R.E. (1986). *Esthetic Composite Bonding - Techniques and Materials*, Blackwell Scientific Publications, England.

Kantorowicz, G.F. (Editor), Cowell, C.R., Curson, I., Kantorowicz, G.F. and Shovelton, D.S. (1985). *Inlays, Crowns and Bridges*, 4th Edn., John Wright & Sons Ltd., Bristol.

Kidd, E.A.M. and Joyston-Bechal, S. (1987). *Essentials of Dental Caries: The Disease and its Management. Dental Practitioner Handbook 31.* John Wright & Sons Ltd., Bristol.

Kidd, E.A.M. and Smith, B.G.N. (1990). *Pickard's Manual of Operative Dentistry*, 6th Edn., Oxford Medical Publications, Oxford.

Messing, J.J. and Stock, C.J.R. (1988). *A Colour Atlas of Endodontics*. Wolfe Medical Publications Ltd., London.

Mohl, N.D., Zarb, G.A., Carlsson, G.E. and Rugh, J.D. (1988). *A Textbook of Occlusion*. Quintessence Publishing Co., Inc., Chicago.

Nicholls, E. (1984). *Endodontics*, 3rd Edn., John Wright & Sons Ltd., Bristol.

Pameijer, J.H.N. (1985). *Periodontal and Occlusal Factors in Crown and Bridge Procedures*. Dental Center for Postgraduate Courses, Amsterdam.

Phillips, R.W. (1991). *Skinner's Science of Dental Materials*, 9th Edn., W.B. Saunders Co., Philadelphia.

Ramfjord, S.P. and Ash, M. (1983). *Occlusion*. 3rd Edn., W.B. Saunders Co., Philadelphia.

Roberts D.H. (1980). *Fixed Bridge Prostheses*. John Wright & Sons Ltd., Bristol.

Shillingburg, H.T., Jacobi, R. and Brackett, S.E. (1987). *Fundamentals of Tooth Preparations - for Cast Metal and Porcelain Restorations*. Quintessence Publishing Co., Inc. Chicago.

Shillingburg, H.T. and Kessler, J.C. (1982). *Restoration of the Endodontically Treated Tooth*. Quintessence Publishing Co., Inc. Chicago.

Smith, B.G.N. (1990). *Planning and Making Crowns and Bridges*, 2nd Edn., Dunitz, London.

Smith, B.G.N., Wright, P.S. and Brown D. (1986). *The Clinical Handling of Dental Materials. Dental Practitioner Handbook* 12, 2nd Edn., John Wright & Sons Ltd., Bristol.

Waite, I.M. and Strahan, J.D. (1990). *A Colour Atlas of Periodontology*, 2nd Edn., Wolfe Publishing Ltd., London.

Bibliography

The following references have been selected from the list of recommended textbooks and other dental literature to complement the text of the Atlas.

Patient assessment and treatment planning

Pameijer, J.H.N. (1985). Chapter 3, Examination, diagnosis and treatment planning. *Periodontal and Occlusal Factors in Crown and Bridge Procedures.*

Hobdell, M. and Elderton, R.J. (Editor) (1990). Chapter 7, Assessment of the patient and principles of treatment planning. *Clinical Dentistry in Health and Disease.* Vol. **3**, The Dentition and Dental Care.

Plaque

Pameijer, J.H.N. (1985). Chapter 6, Plaque control. *Periodontal and Occlusal Factors in Crown and Bridge Procedures.*

Rustogi, N.R., Petrone, D.M., Singh, S.M., Volpe, A.R. and Tavss, E. (1990). Clinical study of a pre-brush rinse and a triclosan/copolymer mouthrinse: Effect on plaque formation. *Am. J. Dent.,* **3**, Special issue, September, S67–S69.

Waite, I.M. and Strahan J.D. (1990). Chapter 9, Control of dental plaque, and Appendix 3, Plaque Indices. *A Colour Atlas of Periodontology.*

Periodontal aspects of conservative dentistry

Leon, A.R. (1977). The periodontium and restorative procedures. A critical review. *J. Oral Rehab.,* **4**, 105.

Pameijer, J.H.N. (1985). Chapter 2, Periodontal and occlusal aspects of crown and bridges. *Periodontal and Occlusal Factors in Crown and Bridge Procedures.*

Ramfjord, S.P. (1974). Periodontal aspects of restorative dentistry. *J. Oral Rehab.,* **1**, 107.

Caries

Elderton, R.J. (1990). Chapter 13, Principles in the management and treatment of dental caries, and Chapter 14, Operative treatment of dental caries. *Clinical Dentistry in Health and Disease,* Vol. **3**, The Dentition and Dental Care.

Mandel, I.D. (1985). Changing patterns of dental caries. *Quint. Int.,* **16**, 81–87.

Kidd, E.A.M. (1984). The diagnosis and management of the early carious lesion in permanent teeth, *Dental Update,* **11**, 69–81.

Kidd, E.A.M. and Joyston-Bechal, S. (1987). Chapter 10, The operative management of caries. *Essentials of Dental Caries.* John Wright, Bristol.

Pulp capping

Stanley, H.R. (1989). Conserving the dental pulp - can it be done, is it worth it? *Oral Surg.,* **68**, 628–639.

Bases and cements

Eccles, J.D. and Green, R.M. (1983). Chapter 6, Linings, cements and dressings. *The Conservation of Teeth.*

Smith, B.G.N., Wright, P.S. and Brown, D. (1986). Chapter 3, Treating caries and other damage to the teeth. *The Clinical Handling of Dental Materials. Dental Practitioner Handbook* **12**.

Principles of cavity preparation

Elderton, R.J. (1984). Cavo-surface angles, amalgam margin angles and occlusal cavity preparations. *Brit. Dent. J.*, **156**, 319–324.

Elderton, R.J. (1984). New approaches to cavity design with special reference to the Class II lesion. *Brit. Dent. J.*, **157**, 421–427.

Elderton, R.J. (1985). Management of early dental caries in fissures with fissure sealant. *Brit. Dent. J.*, **158**, 240–258.

Elderton, R.J. (1985). Assessment and clinical management of early caries in young adults: invasive versus non-invasive methods. *Brit. Dent. J.*, **185**, 440–444.

Elderton, R.J. (1986). Current thinking on cavity design. *Dental Update*, **13**, 113–122.

Hunt, P.R. (1990). Microconservative restorations for approximal caries. *J. Am. Dent. Ass.*, **120**, 37–40.

Kidd, E.A.M. and Smith, B.G.N. (1990). Chapter 3, Principles of cavity design and preparation. *Pickard's Manual of Operative Dentistry*.

Amalgam restorations

Kidd, E.A.M. and Smith, B.G.N. (1990). Chapter 7, Treatment of approximal caries in posterior teeth. *Pickard's Manual of Operative Dentistry*.

Jordan, R.E., Suzuki, M. and Boksman, L. (1985). The new generation of amalgam alloys; clinical considerations. *Dental Clinics of North America*, **29**, 341–358.

Microleakage

Trowbridge, H.O. (1987). Model systems for determining biologic effects of microleakage. *Operative Dentistry*, **12**, 164–172.

Restoration failure

Merrett, M.C.W. and Elderton, R.J. (1984). An in vitro study of restorative treatment decisions and secondary caries. *Brit. Dent. J.*, **157**, 128–133.

Mjor, I.A. (1981). Placement and replacement of restorations. *Operative Dentistry*, **6**, 49–54.

Composite and glass ionomer restorations

Aboush, Y.E.Y. and Jenkins, C.B.G. (1989). The bonding of glass ionomer cement to dental amalgam. *Brit. Dent. J.*, **166**, 255–257.

Barnes, I.E. (1977). The adaptation of composite resins to tooth structure. *Brit. Dent. J.*, **142**, 122, 185, 253, 319.

Hunt, P.R. (1984). A modified Class II cavity preparation for glass ionomer restorative materials. *Quint. Int.*, **10**, 1011–1018.

Jordan, R. (1986). Esthetic composite bonding, *Techniques and Materials*. Blackwell Scientific Publications England.

Kidd, E.A.M. and Smith, B.G.N. (1990). Chapter 6, Treatment of pit and fissure caries; Chapter 8, Treatment of smooth surface caries, erosion-abrasion lesions, and enamel hypoplasia; and Chapter 9, Treatment of approximal caries, trauma, developmental disorders, and discolouration in anterior teeth. *Pickard's Manual of Operative Dentistry*.

McLean, J.W., Prosser, H.J. and Wilson, A.D. (1985). The use of glass-ionomer cements in bonding composite resins to dentine. *Brit. Dent. J.*, **158**, 410–414.

Mount, G.A. (1989). Clinical requirements for a successful 'sandwich' - dentine to glass-ionomer cement to composit resin. *Aust. Dent. J.*, **34**, 259–265.

Taggert, S.E., Pearson, G.J. (1991). The effect of etching on glass polyalkenoate cements. *J. Oral Rehab.*, **18**, 31–42.

Walls, A.W.G., McCabe, J.F. and Murray, J.J. (1988). The polymerisation contraction of visible light activated composite resins. *J. Dent.*, **16**, 177–181.

Welbury, R.R., McCabe, J.F. and Murray, J.J. (1988). Factors affecting the bond strength of composite resin to etched glass ionomer cement. *J. Dent.*, **16**, 188–193.

Wilson, A.D. and McLean, J.W. (1988). *Glass ionomer cements*. Quintessence Publishing Co., Inc. Chicago

Dentine bonding

Causton,B.E., Sefton, J., Some bonding characteristics of a HEMA/maleic acid adhesion promoter. *Brit. Dent. J.*, **167**, 308–311.

Douglas, W.H. (1989). Clinical status of dentine bonding agents. *J. Dent.*, **17**, 209–215.

Pin retention

Wacker, D.R. and Baum, L. (1985). Retentive pins, their use and misuse, p.327, *Dental Clinics of North America* (April).

Winstanley. R.B. (1983). Pinned retention - 10 years on. *Dental Update,* **10**, 246–252.

Gold restorations

Inlays:

Kantorowicz, G.F. (Editor), Cowell, C.R., Curson, I., and Shovelton, D.S. (1985). Chapter 3, Inlay techniques and posterior inlays. *Inlays, Crowns and Bridges.*

Shillingburg, H.T., Jacobi, R. and Brackett, S.E. (1987). Chapter 11, Inlays; Chapter 12, MOD Onlays. *Fundamentals of Tooth Preparations for Cast Metal and Porcelain Restorations.*

Partial veneer crowns:

Kantorowicz, G.F. (Editor), Cowell, C.R., Curson, I., and Shovelton, D.S. (1985). Chapter 8, Three-quarter or partial veneer crowns. *Inlays, Crowns and Bridges.*

Shillingburg, H.T., Jacobi, R. and Brackett, S.E. (1987). Chapter 5, Maxillary posterior three-quarter crowns; Chapter 6, Mandibular posterior three-quarter crowns. *Fundamentals of Tooth Preparations for Cast Metal and Porcelain Restorations.*

Full veneer crowns:

Kantorowicz, G.F. (Editor), Cowell, C.R., Curson, I., and Shovelton, D.S. (1985). Chapter 9, Full veneer crowns on posterior teeth. *Inlays, Crowns and Bridges.*

Shillingburg, H.T., Jacobi, R. and Brackett, S.E. (1987). Chapter 4, Full veneer crowns. *Fundamentals of Tooth Preparations for Cast Metal and Porcelain Restorations.*

Smith, B.G.N. (1990). Chapter 3, Designing crown preparations. *Planning and Making Crowns and Bridges.*

Veneers

McConnell, R.J., Boksman, L. and Gratton, D.R. (1986). Etched porcelain veneers. *Rest. Dent.*, **2,** 124–131.

McLean, J.W. (1988). Ceramics in clinical dentistry. *Brit. Dent. J.*, **164**, 187–194.

Anterior crowns

Jacket crowns:

Kantorowicz, G.F. (Editor), Cowell, C.R., Curson, I., and Shovelton, D.S. (1985). Chapter 6, Anterior crowns. *Inlays, Crowns and Bridges.*

Shillingburg, H.T., Jacobi, R. and Brackett, S.E. (1987). Chapter 15, All-ceramic crowns. *Fundamentals of Tooth Preparations for Cast Metal and Porcelain Restorations.*

Smith, B.G.N. (1990). Chapter 6, Clinical techniques for crown construction. *Planning and Making Crowns and Bridges.*

Post crowns:

Cohen, S. and Burns, R.C. (1991). Chapter 21, Postendodontic restoration. *Pathways of the Pulp*. Wolfe Publishing Ltd., London.

Grundy, J.R. and Glyn Jones, J.C. (1981). Crowning pulpless teeth. *Brit. Dent. J.*, **150**, 307–312, 347–350.

Hunter, A.J. and Flood, A.M. (1989). Restoration of endodontically treated teeth *Aust. Dent. J.*, **34**, 5–12.

Kantorowicz, G.F. (Editor), Cowell, C.R., Curson, I., and Shovelton, D.S. (1985). Chapter 7, Post retained crowns. *Inlays, Crowns and Bridges*.

Ceramics and bonded porcelain

Shillingburg, H.T., Jacobi, R. and Brackett, S.E. (1987). Chapter 13, Anterior porcelain-fused-to-metal crowns; Chapter 14, Posterior porcelain-fused-to-metal crowns. *Fundamentals of Tooth Preparations for Cast Metal and Porcelain Restorations*.

Impression materials

Pameijer, J.H.N. (1985). Chapter 10, Impression procedures for prepared teeth. *Periodontal and Occlusion Factors in Crown and Bridge Procedures*.

Wilson, H.J. (1988). Impression materials. *Brit. Dent. J.*, **164**, 221–225.

Temporary coverage

Braden, M., Causton, B. and Clarke, R.L., (1971). An ethylene imine derivative as a temporary crown and bridge material. *J. Dent. Res.*, **50**, 536–538.

Pameijer, J.H.N. (1985). Chapter 9, Provisional restorations. *Periodontal and Occlusion Factors in Crown and Bridge Procedures*.

Roberts, D.H. (1980). Chapter 16, Impression technique, shade taking and temporary bridges. *Fixed Bridge Prostheses*.

Bridges

Creugers, N.J.H., Snoek, P.A. *et al.*, (1989). Clinical performance of resin bonded bridges. *J. Oral Rehab.*, **16**, 427–436, 521–527.

Kantorowicz, G.F. (Editor), Cowell, C.R., Curson, I., and Shovelton, D.S. (1985). Chapter 11, Principles of bridge design. *Inlays, Crowns and Bridges*.

Roberts, D.H. (1970). The failure of retainers in bridge prostheses: An analysis of 2000 retainers. *Brit. Dent. J.*, **128**, 117–121.

Smith, B.G.N. (1990). Chapter 7, Indications and contraindications for bridges; Chapter 10, Designing and planning bridges. *Planning and Making Crowns and Bridges*.

Tay, W.M. (1986). A classification and assessment of composite retained bridges. *Rest. Dent.*, **2**, 15–22.

Occlusion

Pameijer, J.H.N. (1985). Chapter 5, Occlusion. *Periodontal and Occlusion Factors in Crown and Bridge Procedures*.

Smith, B.G.N. (1990). Chapter 4, Occlusal consideration. *Planning and Making Crowns and Bridges*.

Appendix 1

Procedure for history and examination

History

1. Reason for Attendance
2. Details of Present Complaint (where applicable)
3. Dental History
4. Medical History
5. Family History
6. Personal History

Examination

1. General Assessment – appearance, build, etc.

2. Facial Examination

3. Oral Examination
   (a) Area of present complaint (where applicable)
   (b) General state of the mouth
   (c) Soft tissues
   (d) Periodontal tissues
   (e) Occlusion
   (f) Teeth

4. Special Tests (where applicable)
   (a) Vitality tests
   (b) Radiographs
   (c) Transillumination
   (d) Pulse and temperature
   (e) Study models
   (f) Pathological and biological tests

Appendix 2

Plaque index

The patient hygiene performance index Podshadley and Haley (1968)

1. A disclosing solution is applied to the labial surfaces of the upper first molars, the upper right central incisors and the lower left central incisors and the lingual surfaces of the lower first molars.

   (If the first molar is missing, broken down or crowned, the second molar is substituted. If the central incisor is missing or cannot be used, the adjacent central incisor is substituted.)

2. Each nominated surface is sub-divided mentally into five sections, as indicated below, and examined for stained oil debris or plaque. No stain scores 0, any stain scores 1, for each section. Any tooth surface will therefore have a total score of from 0 to 5.

3. The scores for all surfaces are added together and the sum is divided by the number of surfaces examined (usually 6). This gives the PHP Index.

   e.g.
Upper right first molar	3
Upper right central incisor	2
Upper left first molar	4
Lower left central incisor	3
Lower left first molar	1
Lower right first molar	3
	16

$$PHP = \frac{16}{6} = 2.66$$

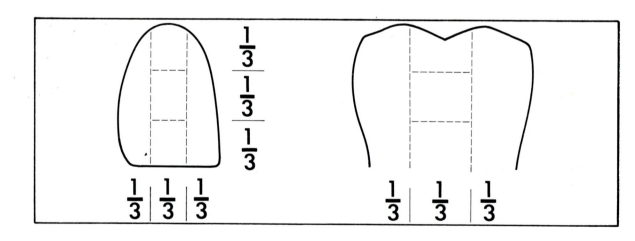

Appendix 3

Alum solution

Alum solution as an adjunct to gingival retraction

Wilson and Tay (1977)

Adrenaline acid tartrate 1%

Sodium metabisulphite 0.1%

In a super saturated solution of:

Potassium aluminium sulphate

Appendix 4

Bases and varnishes

Base materials

Modified zinc/oxide/eugenol cements
Calcium hydroxide
Polycarboxylate cements
Zinc phosphate cements (in association with a subbase)
Ethoxybenzoic acid cements[*]
Glass ionomers[*]

[*]Protection would be required under these cements in deep cavities.

These materials are used:

(a) As protection for the dentine and pulp from chemical or physical irritation

(b) To reduce a deep cavity to appropriate depth for filling

(c) To support undermined enamel

(d) For the elimination of undercuts

Sub-base

Calcium hydroxide in proprietary quick-setting form

Used as an 'indirect pulp cap' to induce pulpal calcification where the floor of a cavity is very close to the pulp. A sub-base may also be applied to the floor of a very deep cavity as protection against possible pulpal irritation from certain bases.

Varnishes

Copal ether varnish
Proprietary varnishes often containing zinc oxide

Used to prevent marginal seepage between an amalgam restoration and the tooth.

Appendix 5

Impression Techniques

Information to be recorded at the chairside

1. The prepared teeth using an elastomeric impression material
2. The opposing teeth using an alginate impression material
3. The occlusal registration

Elastomeric materials available

Addition silicones
Condensation silicones
Polysulphide rubber
Polyether rubber

Indirect techniques

1. Stock tray   (a) Two-stage
                 (b) Single stage

2. Special tray (a) Single stage
                 (b) Two-stage

Appendix 6

Bridge classification

1. Fixed/fixed

A one-piece bridge with the retainers fixed at either end of the pontic

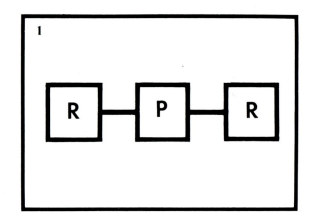

2. Fixed/movable

A two-piece bridge comprising a pontic with a retainer fixed to one end and with a dovetail at the other. The dovetail fits into a slot in the second and independent retainer

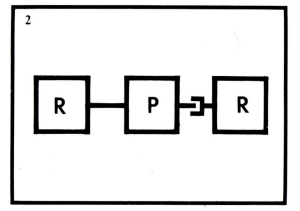

3. Simple cantilever

A bridge where the retainer or retainers are situated at only one end of the pontic

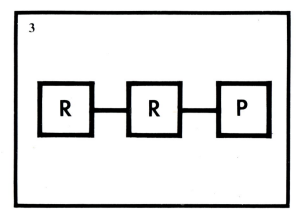

4. Spring cantilever

A bridge where the pontic is connected to the retainer or retainers by means of a bar of metal passing over the palate.

5. Compound bridge

A bridge which combines two or more of the basic designs

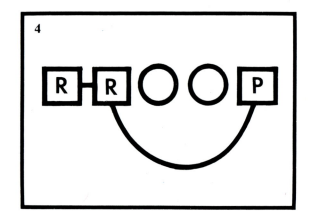

Index

Caption and picture numbers are indicated in bold type.